DOSAGES & SOLUTIONS

A METRIC GUIDE FOR HEALTH PROFESSIONALS

ON

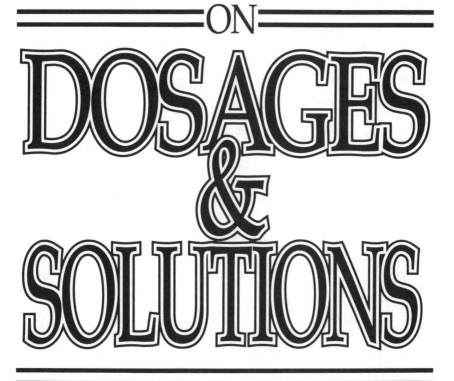

DOSAGES & SOLUTIONS

DEBORAH LYNN DUFF
JOAN MARIE AYLWARD

W.B. Saunders

W.B. Saunders
The Curtis Centre
Independence Square West
Philidelphia, PA 19106

W.B. Saudners Company Canada Limited
55 Horner Avenue
Toronto, Ontario
M8Z 4X6

Canadian Cataloguing in Publication Data

Duff, Deborah, 1955—
    A metric guide for health professionals on dosages and solutions

ISBN 0-9205-1303-4

1.   Drugs - Dosage. 2. Solutions (Pharmacy)
3.   Pharmaceutical arithmetic. 4. Metric system.
I. Aylward, Joan Marie, 1956-   II. Title.

RS57.D83 1984   615.14   C84-099486-9

Cover design/illustrations: Artplus/Brant Cowie
Desktop publishing: Corporate Expressions
Photography: Peter Chan
Production coordination: Francine Geraci

The publisher wishes to thank Glaxo Canada Inc. for making available
samples of Crystapen, Fortaz, Calcium Gluconate and Ventolin for
photographic purposes.

Printed in Canada at The Alger Press

Last digit is the print number: 9 8 7 6 5 4 3 2

PREFACE

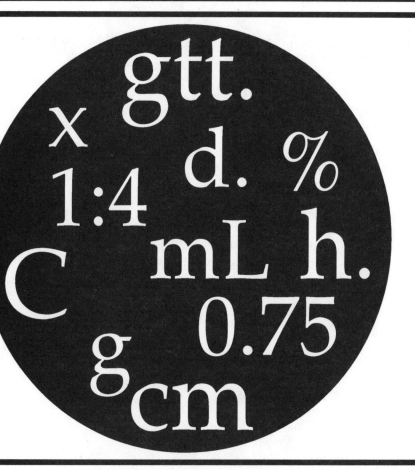

Preface

This programmed text, written by two nursing instructors, is designed primarily for first-year nursing students. It is a valuable reference for other nursing students, graduate nurses, nurses taking a refresher course, and members of various health disciplines, such as pharmacy students.

Other systems of measurement have been deliberately omitted so the student may focus on the International System of Units (SI), which is the official system of measurement in Canada.

The text contains a pretest, an arithmetic review, an introduction to the metric system, calculation of dosages and solutions, a post-test, and appendices. Each chapter outlines relevant objectives.

The pretest allows for individual pacing and ongoing self-evaluation of the basic arithmetic skills.

The arithmetic review encompasses the necessary mathematical concepts. The desired outcome of this review is for the individual to progress systematically from basic arithmetic skills to more difficult concepts.

Chapter 3 outlines the metric system and provides the necessary instruction to allow the individual to use it effectively.

Chapters 4 through 8 concentrate on specific areas relevant to dosage and solution calculation. A standard formula is used consistently, where applicable. This edition uses proportions as an alternate formula. This method has been included to relate a familiar concept to the often confusing calculation of dosages and solutions.

It is hoped that mature students and those who encounter difficulty remembering numerous formulae will find this method helpful.

The post-test is a cumulative review of all the concepts detailed in previous chapters. This includes basic arithmetic and calculations for dosages and solutions.

The appendices are quick, easy references that include answers to all problems, a collection of terminology, metric base units, equivalencies relevant to the three systems of measurement, abbreviations and symbols, children's formulae, insulins, and a review of all formulae used throughout the text.

When this revised edition was originally planned, the chapter on solutions was to be omitted. After discussion with pharmacists who emphasized the importance of solution preparation for pharmacy students, the chapter was retained and revised. It was intentionally placed as the final chapter of calculations so that it may be omitted without disrupting the progress of concepts. Nurses or other health professionals may use this chapter as a reference, when required.

The text is designed to introduce each new concept, accompanied by practical examples, including both adult and child dosages. Necessary formulae are stated with detailed examples of the work.

Individuals may test and evaluate their understanding of new material by completing the practice problems following each new concept. Answers to all problems are provided in the appendices. Problems should be worked completely before referring to the answers. Those encountering difficulty solving problems should review the appropriate sections.

Because many problems arise from poor mathematical skills, it is strongly suggested that calculators not be used. Keep in mind the possibility that calculators may not be available when dosage problems occur.

With the ever-present need for safety, the individual must first understand the concepts of basic mathematics. Having acquired this skill, the individual will demonstrate the ability to prepare and administer medications safely.

To the Instructor:

This text may be used for self-instruction, organized classroom teaching, or for remedial practice. Not all instructors may choose to cover each area included.

This edition contains a pretest of 100 questions, many of which are new. These questions test each concept beginning with the simple concept and progressing to the more difficult. This design permits the instructor to assess the individual's problem area, whether it be mathematical or conceptual. The post-test includes 200 questions, testing all concepts. Both tests can be used for class assignments, quizzes, or as extra practice problems.

To assure safety in the preparation and administration of medications, a minimum grade of 80% is recommended.

This text is designed with one goal in mind: that the basic mathematical skills be understood and mastered. It is for this reason that advanced skills required for safe medication preparation and administration have been omitted.

The response to the first edition of this *Canadian Metric Guide* was overwhelming. All feedback received was reviewed. Considerable changes, some relevant to the feedback received, have been made in this new edition.

Changes include the addition of Roman numeral conversions, more diagrams, such as tablets, medicine cups, insulin syringes, and outlined formulae. All medications are now identified by their generic and trade names.

New material has been added, including chapter objectives, the dates in metric, heparin and aminophylline infusions, ratios, and children's formulae.

A major change involved breaking Chapter 4 in the first edition into five new chapters. These chapters progress through different dosage and solution calculations. This edition presents these concepts in a more organized sequence. Concepts are now immediately followed by specific examples.

The post-test is more comprehensive. Changes to the appendices include new definitions and abbreviations, insulins, and body surface area (BSA) formulae, as well as obsolete children's formulae.

We anticipate your valued feedback on our new edition. We hope that, by responding to your individual suggestions, we have helped make this second edition even more suitable to your needs.

Thank you,

Deborah Lynn Duff, B.N., R.N.
Joan Marie J. Aylward, R.N., B.N.
St. Clare's Mercy Hospital
School of Nursing
St. John's, Newfoundland

Acknowledgments

Revision of a text would not be possible without the continued feedback of its many users. We wish to thank all instructors, librarians, pharmacists, and other health professionals who offered their valuable comments.

It is with our appreciation that we continue to acknowledge all those nursing students who have shown us their great need for this basic dosage and solutions text. It is not only you who learn from us—but us from you.

Special Thanks

To Linda Hensman, Pharm D., Director of Pharmacy, St. Clare's Mercy Hospital, St. John's, Newfoundland—we thank you for your time, interest, and valuable material.

To Sheila Howell, R.N., Diabetic Instructor, St. Clare's Mercy Hospital, St. John's, Newfoundland—we thank you for your current update on insulins.

To Brian Healy, Ph.C., Past President, Newfoundland Pharmaceutical Association—we thank you for your information on the presentation of pediatric orders.

To Merlee Steele-Rodway, R.N., staff graduate, Intensive Care Unit, Janeway Children's Hospital, St. John's, Newfoundland— we thank you for your information on practical pediatric examples.

To Jane Grant, secretary, St. Clare's Mercy Hospital School of Nursing—we thank you for arranging the safe transport, on a moment's notice, of the revisions as they were completed.

To our many friends and family—we thank you for your interest, support, and love.

To Sonny (Gordon Aylward)—we thank you for your long-distance support and encouragement.

To John, who improved his typing skills making all those "revisions to the revisions"—we never would have made it without you: THANKS.

To Dad for being there.

To our Moms, Thank you for all the babysitting, etc., etc., etc. What more can we say?

To our children: John, Alison, Maria, and Jenna—the book is finished; we will have that "time" for you now.

Table of Contents

CHAPTER 1: PRETEST

XL

0.7

ROMAN NUMERALS

4:11

9 X 0.1 =

1/8

V $\overline{SS}$

$\dfrac{2/15}{20}$

divisor

25 - 2 5/6 ==

mixed numbers

numerator

5 2/7 =

decimals

x = 33

3/9 + 7/10 =

improper fractions

%

CHAPTER 1

Objectives

1. The student will identify any conceptual or practical weaknesses in basic mathematical skills, advancing from simple to complex.

2. The student will seek additional guidance in any demonstrated areas of weaknesses.

PRELIMINARY ASSESSMENT

Answer the following questions. Show any work needed to achieve the final answer. See Appendix A for answers to questions 1 through 100.

Convert the following Arabic numerals to Roman numerals:

1.   8   2.   14

3.   16   4.   25

Convert the following Roman numerals to Arabic numerals:

5.   xii   6.   XVII

7.   xv   8.   XXIV......

Convert the following improper fractions to whole or mixed numbers:

9. $7/3$ 10. $5/5$

Convert the following mixed numbers to improper fractions:

11. $2^1/_7$ 12. $3^1/_4$

Convert the following complex fractions to proper or improper fractions:

13. $\dfrac{2/11}{6}$ 14. $\dfrac{9}{3/7}$

Add the following fractions:

15. $2/_{11} + 5/_{11} =$ 16. $^1/_5 + ^2/_5 =$

Add the following fractions and reduce to lowest terms:

17. $^1/_2 + ^3/_4 =$ 18. $^3/_4 + ^6/_7 =$

Add the following mixed numbers and reduce to lowest terms:

19. $1^5/_6 + 3^2/_3 =$ 20. $2^2/_{10} + 4^7/_8 =$

Subtract the following fractions:

21. $3/7 - 2/7 =$ 22. $11/19 - 6/19 =$

Subtract the following fractions and reduce to lowest terms:

23. $5/6 - 1/2 =$ 24. $4/5 - 2/3 =$

Subtract the following mixed numbers and reduce to lowest terms:

25. $4\,8/9 - 2\,1/27 =$ 26. $4\,6/7 - 3\,1/3 =$

Multiply the following fractions:

27. $1/4 \times 1/3 =$ 28. $1/11 \times 5/3 =$

Multiply the following fractions and reduce to lowest terms:

29. $7/8 \times 2/3 =$ 30. $9/10 \times 2/5 =$

Multiply the following mixed numbers and reduce to lowest terms:

31. $2\,1/2 \times 3\,1/4 =$ 32. $1\,5/16 \times 1\,2/3 =$

Divide the following fractions:

33. $1/2 \div 7 =$ 34. $3/7 \div 5 =$

Divide the following fractions and reduce to lowest terms:

35. $5/8 \div 1/7 =$ 36. $7/8 \div 3/4 =$

Divide the following mixed numbers and reduce to lowest terms:

37. $6\,1/2 \div 3\,1/2 =$ 38. $7\,2/8 \div 3\,1/4 =$

39. $10\,1/2 \div 4\,3/4 =$ 40. $7\,2/5 \div 3\,1/4 =$

Convert the following fractions to decimal fractions. Carry to the third decimal place:

41. $^2/_{10}$ 42. $^3/_{1\,000}$

43. $^6/_{25}$ 44. $^1/_6$

Convert the following decimal fractions to improper fractions and reduce to lowest terms:

45. 0.16   46. 0.3

47. 0.645   48. 0.72

Add the following decimal fractions:

49. 0.349 + 0.024 6 =   50. 7.543 + 2.909 =

51. 0.239 + 0.005 =   52. 5.255 + 0.916 2 =

Subtract the following decimal fractions:

53. 0.949 - 0.321 =   54. 2.0 - 0.004 18 =

55. 0.007 5 - 0.000 39 =   56. 27.363 - 10.154 =

Multiply the following decimal fractions:

57. 50.0 x 0.001 =   58. 7.3 x 0.01 =

59. 0.08 x 0.1 =   60. 29.32 x 1.0 =

61. 9.753 x 10.3 =   62. 0.020 5 x 27.4 =

Divide the following decimal fractions. Carry to the third decimal place:

63. 0.765 ÷ 0.001 =   64. 273.4 ÷ 0.01 =

65. 3.586 ÷ 0.1 =   66. 102.97 ÷ 1.0 =

67. 6.001 ÷ 5.9 =   68. 14.0 ÷ 0.003 5 =

Convert the following percentages to common fractions or whole numbers:

69. $^1/_5\%$ 70. 33%

Convert the following percentages to decimal fractions:

71.   10%   72. $^4/_5$%

Convert the following fractions to percentages:

73. $^7/_{35}$ 74. $^1/_{100}$

Convert the following decimal fractions to percentages:

75.   0.6   76.   2.08

Convert the following proper fractions to ratios and reduce to lowest terms:

77. $^5/_9$ 78. $^{24}/_{36}$

Convert the following decimal fractions to ratios and reduce to lowest terms:

79.   0.565   80.   0.40

Convert the following ratios to fractions and reduce to lowest terms:

81.   10 : 100   82.   5 : 60

Convert the following ratios to decimal fractions:

83.   6 : 7   84.   31 : 9

Convert the following percentages to ratios and reduce to lowest terms:

85.   25%   86.   57%

Convert the following ratios to percentages:

87.   25 : 100   88.   9 : 25

Calculate the value of X and reduce to lowest terms:

89. $20 : 100 :: X : 200$

90. $1/2 : 5/8 :: X : 2/3$

91. $0.002 : 5 :: X : 10$

92. $5 : X :: 10 : 300$

93. The upper number of a fraction is the _____.

94. The lower number of a fraction is the _____.

95. Write the following mixed number: twenty-seven and eight hundredths: _____.

96. When the upper number of a fraction is larger than the lower, it is referred to as a(n) _____.

97. L.C.D. is an abbreviation for _____.

98. Which decimal fraction is the largest: 0.05 or 0.009? _____.

99. Write the following ratio: nineteen is to fifty-seven. _____.

100. Write the following proportion: eleven is to two as thirty-three is to six._____.

CHAPTER 2:
ARITHMETIC REVIEW

XL

0.7

ROMAN NUMERALS

4:11

9 X 0.1=

1/8

V $\overline{SS}$

$\dfrac{2/15}{20}$

divisor

25 - 2 5/6=

numerator

mixed numbers

5 2/7=

decimals

x= 33

3/9 + 7/10 =

improper fractions

%

CHAPTER 2

Objectives

1. The student will demonstrate an understanding of basic mathematical concepts.

2. The student will demonstrate the ability to solve basic mathematical problems accurately.

ARABIC AND ROMAN NUMERALS

There are two numeral systems health professionals may encounter: Arabic and Roman. The most common is the Arabic system.

The Arabic system uses the numbers 0 through 9. Values less than 0 are written as proper or decimal fractions. (See Appendix J for definitions of unfamiliar terms.)

EXAMPLE: 1/2 or 0.5

The Roman system may occasionally be used by physicians to prescribe medications. This system uses letters. The numbers 1 through 100 will be reviewed for application by health professionals. Figure 2–1 lists the basic letters in the Roman system and their Arabic equivalent.

ROMAN		ARABIC
ss	s̄s̄	1/2
I	(i)	1
V	(v)	5
X	(x)	10
L	(l)	50
C	(c)	100
D	(d)	500
M	(m)	1 000

Figure 2–1:   Basic Roman and Arabic equivalents.

To CONVERT ARABIC NUMERALS to ROMAN NUMERALS:

A.   Capital letters are generally used. Lower-case letters are used when expressing dosages or working with the apothecary system of measurement. (Figure 2–1.)

   EXAMPLE: On a prescription, 5 would be written as v, not V.

B.   Place the largest valued letters on the left and the smallest valued letters on the right.

   EXAMPLE: 15 would be written as xv, NOT vx.

C. A letter can be used a maximum of three consecutive times. When a smaller valued letter is to the left of a larger valued letter, the numeral corresponding with the smaller valued letter is subtracted from the numeral corresponding with the larger valued letter.

EXAMPLES: 3 would be written as iii or III.

---

4 would be written as iv or IV, NOT iiii or IIII.

D. Fractions are expressed in the same way as the Arabic system with one exception: $1/2$ = ss or $\overline{ss}$

EXAMPLE: $5\,1/2$ = vss or v$\overline{ss}$

NOTE: See Appendix B for answers to questions in this chapter.

Convert the following Arabic numerals to Roman numerals:

1. 2   2. $9\,1/2$
3. 13   4.   59
5. 21

To CONVERT ROMAN NUMERALS to ARABIC NUMERALS:

A. The smallest numerals are added to the largest and identical numerals are added.

EXAMPLE: xxviii in the Arabic system is

x = 10

v = 5

i = 1

10 + 10 + 5 + 1 + 1 + 1 = 28

B. When a lesser numeral follows a greater numeral, the numerals are added.

    EXAMPLE: LX in the Arabic system is

        L = 50

        X = 10

        50 + 10 = 60

C. When a greater numeral follows a lesser numeral, the numerals are subtracted.

    EXAMPLE: XL in the Arabic system is

        X = 10

        L = 50

        50 - 10 = 40

D. When a lesser numeral is between a series of numerals, the lesser numeral is read with the numeral following it.

    EXAMPLE: LXXIV in the Arabic system is

        L = 50

        X = 10

        I = 1

        V = 5

        50 + 10 + 10 + (5 - 1) =

        50 + 10 + 10 + 4 = 74

Convert the following Roman numerals to Arabic numerals:

6.   xii   7.   VL

8.   LV   9   CXIV

10.   XXX$\overline{ss}$

FRACTIONS

A *fraction* represents the division of a whole number. It is expressed by using a numerator and a denominator.

The *numerator*, or the number above the line, is the *dividend*. It indicates how many parts of the divided unit are taken.

The *denominator*, or number below the line, is the *divisor*. It indicates how many parts the whole unit is divided into.

The numerator and denominator are called *terms* of a fraction.

> *EXAMPLE:*   Three-quarters would be written as:
>
> $3/4$ or $\dfrac{3}{4}$ where 3 is the numerator
>
> where 4 is the denominator
>
> 3 and 4 are the terms

A *proper fraction* is a fraction in which the numerator is smaller than the denominator. It can also be referred to as a simple or common fraction.

EXAMPLES: $1/2$, $3/4$, $9/11$

An *improper fraction* is a fraction in which the numerator is equal to or larger than the denominator.

EXAMPLES: $2/2$, $7/5$, $24/19$

A *mixed number* is a fraction preceded by a whole number.

EXAMPLES: $1\,1/2$, $7\,5/8$, $13\,2/3$

A *complex fraction* is a fraction in which there is a fraction in the numerator, denominator, or both.

EXAMPLES: $\dfrac{1/4}{10}$, $\dfrac{5}{1/2}$, $\dfrac{1/3}{1/6}$

CONVERSIONS

To CONVERT an IMPROPER FRACTION to a WHOLE NUMBER or MIXED NUMBER:

A. Divide the numerator by the denominator.

B. Place the remainder over the denominator.

EXAMPLES: $7/2 =$

$$7 \div 2 =$$

$$2 \overline{)7}^{\,3}$$

$$\frac{6}{1}$$

$$= 3\ 1/2$$

_____

$3/3 =$

$$3 \div 3 =$$

$$3 \overline{)3}^{\,1}$$

$$= 1$$

To CONVERT a MIXED NUMBER to an IMPROPER FRACTION:

A. Multiply the whole number by the denominator of the fraction.

B. Add this total to the numerator of the fraction.

C. Place the total over the denominator of the fraction.

EXAMPLE: $3\,^5/_6 = \dfrac{(3 \times 6) + 5}{6} = \,^{23}/_6$

To CONVERT a COMPLEX FRACTION to a WHOLE NUMBER, PROPER FRACTION, or IMPROPER FRACTION:

A. Divide the numerator by the denominator.

B. To divide a number by a fraction, invert the numerator and denominator of the divisor and multiply the numerators together and the denominators together.

EXAMPLES: $\dfrac{5}{1/3} = 5 \div \,^1/_3 = 5 \times \,^3/_1 = 15$

$\dfrac{1/4}{10} = \,^1/_4 \div 10 = \,^1/_4 \times \,^1/_{10} = \,^1/_{40}$

$\dfrac{1/12}{1/3} = \,^1/_{12} \div \,^1/_3 = \,^1/_{12} \times \,^3/_1 = \,^3/_{12} = \,^1/_4$

$\dfrac{5}{2/17} = 5 \div \,^2/_{17} = 5 \times \,^{17}/_2 = \,^{85}/_2$

Convert the following improper fractions to whole or mixed numbers:

11. $^{19}/_{19} =$ 12. $^{22}/_2 =$

13. $^8/_5 =$ 14. $^{89}/_{11} =$

15. $^{43}/_{15} =$

Convert the following mixed numbers to improper fractions:

16. $3\,^1/_7 =$ 17. $2\,^1/_8 =$

18. $11\,^1/_2 =$ 19. $7\,^1/_6 =$

20. $5\,^2/_6 =$

Convert the following complex fractions to whole numbers, proper fractions, or improper fractions:

21. $\dfrac{1/2}{2} =$ 22. $\dfrac{1/7}{12} =$

23. $\dfrac{1/5}{1/9} =$ 24. $\dfrac{12/14}{20/51} =$

25. $\dfrac{28}{1/4} =$

REDUCING TO LOWEST TERMS

Reducing a fraction to lowest terms does not change the value of the fraction. The fraction is stated with proportionally smaller numbers. The numerator and denominator are divided by the same whole number, known as the *largest common divisor*. This number is the largest number that will divide evenly into the numerator and denominator.

> *EXAMPLE:* $^6/_{12}$
>
> 6 is the largest common divisor.
>
> $\dfrac{6 \div 6}{12 \div 6} = \dfrac{1}{2} = {}^1/_2$

FINDING THE LOWEST COMMON DENOMINATOR

The *lowest common denominator (LCD)* is the smallest number into which all denominators found in a group of fractions are divisible. To add or subtract fractions, all denominators must be common. Therefore, it may be necessary to convert a group of fractions to the lowest common denominator.

To CONVERT FRACTIONS to the LOWEST COMMON DENOMINATOR:

A. Divide the lowest common denominator by the denominator of the fraction.

B. Multiply the answer by the numerator of the same fraction.

C.   Place the result over the lowest common denominator.

EXAMPLE: $1/2 + 3/4 =$

The LCD is 4.

$1/2 = (4 \div 2) \times 1 = 2 \times 1 = 2/4$

$3/4 = (4 \div 4) \times 3 = 1 \times 3 = 3/4$

$2/4 + 3/4 = 5/4 = 1 1/4$

Reduce the following fractions to lowest terms:

26. $10/20 =$ 27. $15/60 =$

28. $\dfrac{16}{2/3} =$ 29. $183/29 =$

30. $62/19 =$

ADDING FRACTIONS

To ADD FRACTIONS if the denominators are common:

A.   Add the numerators.

B.   Place the total number over the common denominator.

C.   Reduce to lowest terms.

EXAMPLES: $1/5 + 3/5 = 4/5$

$1/6 + 1/6 = 2/6 = 1/3$

To ADD FRACTIONS if the denominators are different:

A.   Convert the fractions to the lowest common denominator.

B.   Add the numerators.

C.   Place the total over the common denominator.

D.   Reduce to lowest terms.

EXAMPLE: $1/3 + 1/6 =$

The lowest common denominator is 6.

$2/6 = 1/6 = 3/6 = 1/2$

To ADD MIXED NUMBERS:

A.   Convert each mixed number to an improper fraction.

B.   Convert the fractions to the lowest common denominator.

C.   Add the numerators.

D.   Place the total over the common denominator.

E.   Reduce to lowest terms.

EXAMPLE: $1\,1/2 + 2\,1/3 =$

$3/2 + 7/3 =$

$9/6 + 14/6 = 23/6 = 3\,5/6$

Add the following fractions and reduce to lowest terms:

31.	$1/7 + 2/7 =$	32.	$3/4 + 1/5 =$
33.	$6\,1/3 + 3\,1/6 =$	34.	$10\,1/9 + 12\,1/6 =$
35.	$21\,10/11 + 14\,1/6 =$		

SUBTRACTING FRACTIONS

To SUBTRACT FRACTIONS if the denominators are common:

A.   Subtract the numerator of the number on the right from the numerator of the number on the left.

B.   Place the remaining number over the common denominator.

C.   Reduce to lowest terms.

EXAMPLES: $7/8 - 2/8 = 5/8$

$3/4 - 1/4 = 2/4 = 1/2$

To SUBTRACT FRACTIONS if the denominators are different:

A. Convert the fractions to the lowest common denominator.

B. Subtract the numerator of the fraction on the right from the numerator of the fraction on the left.

C. Place the remaining number over the common denominator.

D. Reduce to lowest terms.

> *EXAMPLE:* $5/12 - 1/4 =$
>
> The lowest common denominator is 12.
>
> $5/12 - 3/12 = 2/12 = 1/6$

To SUBTRACT MIXED NUMBERS:

A. Convert each mixed number to an improper fraction.

B. Convert the fractions to the lowest common denominator.

C. Subtract the numerators.

D. Place the total over the common denominator.

E. Reduce to lowest terms.

> *EXAMPLE:* $2 1/4 - 1 1/3 =$
>
> $9/4 - 4/3 =$
>
> $27/12 - 16/12 = 11/12$

Subtract the following fractions and reduce to lowest terms:

36. $^{11}/_{12} - ^{4}/_{12} =$ 37. $^{4}/_{5} - ^{1}/_{6} =$

38. $3^{2}/_{7} - 1^{9}/_{10} =$ 39. $7^{1}/_{5} - 3^{1}/_{7} =$

40. $17^{1}/_{4} - 13^{2}/_{5} =$

MULTIPLYING FRACTIONS

To MULTIPLY FRACTIONS:

A. Reduce all fractions to lowest terms.

B. Cross cancel where possible.

C. Multiply all numerators.

D. Multiply all denominators.

E. Place the total of the numerators over the total of the denominators.

F. Reduce to lowest terms.

EXAMPLES: $^{3}/_{4} \times ^{10}/_{12} =$

$^{3}/_{4} \times ^{5}/_{6} =$

$^{1}\!\!\!3/_{4} \times ^{5}/\!\!\!6\,2 = \dfrac{1 \times 5}{4 \times 2} = ^{5}/_{8}$

_____

$^{6}/_{8} \times ^{5}/_{9} =$

$^{3}/_{4} \times ^{5}/_{9} =$

$^{1}\!\!\!3/_{4} \times ^{5}/\!\!\!9\,3 = \dfrac{1 \times 5}{4 \times 3} = ^{5}/_{12}$

To MULTIPLY MIXED NUMBERS:

A. Convert each mixed number to an improper fraction.

B.   Reduce all fractions to lowest terms.

C.   Cross cancel where possible.

D.   Multiply all numerators.

E.   Multiply all denominators.

F.   Place the total of the numerators over the total of the denominators.

G.   Reduce to lowest terms.

> *EXAMPLE:* $2^1/_3 \times 4^1/_5 =$
>
> $^7/_3 \times {}^{21}/_5 =$
>
> $^7/_{3\,1} \times {}^7{}^{21}\!/_5 = \dfrac{7 \times 7}{1 \times 5} = {}^{49}/_5 = 9^4/_5$

Multiply the following fractions and reduce to lowest terms:

41. $^7/_6 \times {}^4/_5 =$ 42. $^2/_{11} \times {}^3/_{17} =$

43. $13^4/_6 \times 2^1/_3 =$ 44. $25 \times {}^3/_4 =$

45. $6^1/_9 \times 14^1/_{13} =$

DIVIDING FRACTIONS

To DIVIDE a FRACTION by a FRACTION:

A.   Invert the divisor.

B.   Cross cancel where possible.

C.   Multiply the fractions.

D.   Reduce to lowest terms.

> *EXAMPLE:* $^3/_4 \div {}^1/_2 = {}^3/_4 \times {}^2/_1 =$
>
> $^3/_{4\,2} \times {}^1{}^2\!/_1 = \dfrac{3 \times 1}{2 \times 1} = {}^3/_2 = 1^1/_2$

To DIVIDE MIXED NUMBERS:

A. Convert all mixed numbers to improper fractions.

B. Invert the divisor.

C. Cross cancel where possible.

D. Multiply the fractions.

E. Reduce to lowest terms.

EXAMPLE: $2^1/5 \div 3^1/2 =$

$^{11}/5 \div ^7/2 =$

$^{11}/5 \times ^2/7 = ^{22}/35$

Divide the following fractions and reduce to lowest terms:

46. $^3/7 \div ^1/3 =$ 47. $^1/2 \div ^1/11 =$

48. $9^3/16 \div 4^2/7 =$ 49. $32^1/3 \div 1^1/4 =$

50. $2^4/9 \div ^1/6 =$

DECIMAL FRACTIONS

A fraction is normally expressed as a numerator over a denominator. However, when the numerator has been divided by the denominator, the result is a *decimal number*.

To CONVERT an IMPROPER FRACTION to a DECIMAL NUMBER:

Divide the numerator by the denominator.

EXAMPLE: $^1/4 =$

$$
\begin{array}{r}
0.25 \\
4\overline{)1.00} \\
\underline{8\,0} \\
20 \\
\underline{2\,0} \\
0
\end{array}
$$

0.25 is a decimal number.

In a decimal fraction, the denominator is 10 or some multiple of 10. The denominator is indicated by a decimal sign, or a period, referred to as the *decimal*. Whole numbers are written to the left of the decimal. Fractions are written to the right of the decimal.

To CONVERT a DECIMAL NUMBER to an IMPROPER FRACTION:

A.   Move the decimal to the right to make a whole number.

B.   Write the whole number as the numerator.

C.   Multiply 1 by 10 for each place the decimal is moved to give 10 or a multiple of 10 (or for each place the decimal is moved add a zero to 1).

D.   Write the result as the denominator.

EXAMPLE: 0.37 =

$$\frac{37}{100}$$ The decimal is moved two places.
1 x 10 x 10 = 100
37   is the numerator
100   is the denominator

Decimal numbers are read from left to right. Each digit, including the decimal, is stated.

EXAMPLE: 3.456 is read as:

three, decimal, four, five, six.

Some decimal numbers are indefinite. These numbers are generally rounded off to a specified number of decimal places. If the next number is 5 or greater, the previous number increases by 1.

EXAMPLES: $1/9 =$

$1 \div 9 = 0.111\ 1$

0.111 1 rounded to the third decimal place =
0.111.

$4/11 =$

$4 \div 11 = 0.363\ 6$

0.363 6 rounded to the third decimal place =
0.364.

Convert the following fractions to decimal numbers. Carry to the third decimal place:

51. $1/8 =$ 52. $7/15 =$

53. $3/9 =$ 54. $5\,1/5 =$

55. $11\,7/21 =$

Convert the following decimal numbers to proper fractions. Reduce to lowest terms:

56. $0.742 =$ 57. $0.07 =$

58. $0.46 =$ 59. $0.19 =$

60. $0.9 =$

ADDING AND SUBTRACTING DECIMAL NUMBERS

To ADD or SUBTRACT DECIMAL NUMBERS:

A. Place all decimals in vertical alignment.

B. Fill in columns by adding zeroes.

C. Complete the problem as indicated by the symbol.

D. Place the decimal in the answer directly below the decimals in the problem.

E. If the answer results in a decimal number of less than one, place a zero to the left of the decimal.

EXAMPLES: 3.41 + 6.151 + 0.614 =

$$
\begin{array}{r}
3.410 \\
6.151 \\
+\quad 0.614 \\
\hline
10.175
\end{array}
$$

10.452 - 9.542 =

$$
\begin{array}{r}
10.452 \\
-\quad 9.542 \\
\hline
0.910
\end{array}
$$

Add the following decimal numbers:

61. 2.148 + 1.961 =   62. 0.047 3 + 0.001 =

63. 0.001 4 + 0.045 6 =   64. 69.040 + 3.001 4 =

65. 591.16 + 76.35 =

Subtract the following decimal numbers:

66. 0.009 27 - 0.004 =   67. 12.741 - 11.992 =

68. 40.24 - 30.952 =   69. 1 453.4 - 959.412 =

70. 53.040 1 - 49.62 =

MULTIPLYING DECIMAL NUMBERS

Decimal numbers are multiplied the same as any multiplication problem. It is important to ensure correct placement of the decimal in the final answer.

To MULTIPLY DECIMAL NUMBERS:

A. Count the number of places to the right of the decimal in the *multiplicand.*

B. Count the number of places to the right of the decimal in the *multiplier.*

C. Add both.

D. Using this total, count from right to left to place the decimal correctly in the total of the equation.

> EXAMPLE: 18.96 x 1.41 =
>
> | | |
> |---|---|
> | 18.96 | There are two places to the right |
> | x 1.41 | of the decimal on both lines. |
> | 1896 | |
> | 7584 | |
> | 1896 | |
> | 26.733 6 | Decimal is moved four places to the left. |

Multiply the following decimal numbers.

71.	0.46 x 1.21 =		72.	5.15 x 11.06 =
73.	2.46 x 8.71 =		74.	27.409 x 11.3 =
75.	0.004 2 x 0.002 9 =		76.	19.079 x 10.1 =
77.	85.051 x 20.006 4 =		78.	3.197 x 2.0 =
79.	131.75 x 0.21 =		80.	21.967 x 14.304 =

DIVIDING DECIMAL NUMBERS

Decimal numbers are divided the same way as any division problem. The decimal is considered before calculation.

To DIVIDE DECIMAL NUMBERS:

A. Move the decimal in the divisor to make a whole number.

B. Move the decimal in the dividend the same number of places.

C. The decimal in the answer is located directly above the decimal in the dividend.

D. Zeroes may be added to the dividend to extend the number of places after the decimal.

EXAMPLE: 96.562 ÷ 4.1 =

$$
\begin{array}{r}
23.551 \\
41\,\overline{)965.620} \\
\underline{82} \\
145 \\
\underline{123} \\
226 \\
\underline{205} \\
212 \\
\underline{205} \\
70 \\
\underline{41} \\
29
\end{array}
$$

Divide the following decimal numbers. Carry to the third decimal place.

81.	1.75 ÷ 0.32 =	82.	20.16 ÷ 0.04 =
83.	10.5 ÷ 2.6 =	84.	72.34 ÷ 16.37 =
85.	84.0 ÷ 3.151 =	86.	100.404 ÷ 51.2 =
87.	712.61 ÷ 49.39 =	88.	17.3 ÷ 0.09 =
89.	42.11 ÷ 38.1 =	90.	68.14 ÷ 7.33 =

MULTIPLYING AND DIVIDING BY 10
or multiples of 10 (100, 1 000, 10 000, etc.)

In multiplication and division of decimals by 10 or multiples of 10, there is no need to complete the problem in the long standard form. A shorter method relocates the position of the decimal.

To MULTIPLY:

A. Move the decimal in the multiplicand as many places to the right as there are zeroes in the multiplier.

B. Zeroes may be added to the multiplicand if required.

 EXAMPLES: 0.3 x 10 = 3.0

 ———————————————————————

 0.3 x 100 = 30.0

 ———————————————————————

 0.3 x 1 000 = 300.0

To DIVIDE:

A. Move the decimal in the dividend as many places to the left as there are zeroes in the divisor.

B. Zeroes may be added to the dividend if required.

 EXAMPLES: 20.9 ÷ 10 = 2.09

 ———————————————————————

 0.078 ÷ 100 = 0.000 78

 ———————————————————————

 50 297.03 ÷ 1 000 = 50.297 03

Multiply the following:

91.	0.032 x 100 =	92.	2.714 x 10 =
93.	0.004 7 x 1 000 =	94.	17.321 x 1 000 =
95.	127.69 x 10 =	96.	68.88 x 100 =
97.	0.104 9 x 1 000 =	98.	1 001.04 x 100 =
99.	783.33 x 100 =	100.	467.03 x 10 =

Divide the following:

101.	2.304 ÷ 100 =	102.	0.029 ÷ 10 =

103.	15.623 ÷ 1 000 =		104.	36.920 ÷ 100 =
105.	0.001 ÷ 1 000 =		106.	1 066.7 ÷ 100 =
107.	42.007 ÷ 100 =		108.	377.047 ÷ 10 =
109.	10.891 ÷ 1 000 =		110.	1 632.41 ÷ 100 =

MULTIPLYING AND DIVIDING BY 0.1
or multiples of 0.1 (0.01, 0.001, 0.000 1, etc.)

In multiplication and division of decimals by 0.1 or multiples of 0.1, there is no need to complete the problem in the long standard form. Calculation is simply a matter of moving the position of the decimal.

To MULTIPLY:

A. Move the decimal in the multiplicand as many places to the left as there are zeroes in the multiplier.

B. Zeroes may be added to the multiplicand if required.

EXAMPLES: 1.5 x 0.1 = 0.15

150.41 x 0.01 = 1.504 1

25.36 x 0.001 = 0.025 36

To DIVIDE:

A. Move the decimal in the dividend as many places to the right as there are zeroes in the divisor.

B. Zeroes may be added to the dividend if required.

EXAMPLES: 10 ÷ 0.1 = 100

258 ÷ 0.01 = 25 800

947.590 ÷ 0.001 = 947 590

Multiply the following:

111.	0.01 x 0.1 =		112.	10.62 x 0.01 =
113.	156.34 x 0.001 =		114.	0.003 6 x 0.000 1 =
115.	17.19 x 0.1 =		116.	156.11 x 0.01 =
117.	369.90 x 0.001 =		118.	46.03 x 0.000 1 =
119.	0.007 1 x 0.1 =		120.	189.21 x 0.01 =

Divide the following:

121.	0.42 ÷ 0.1 =		122.	10.26 ÷ 0.01 =
123.	3.14 ÷ 0.001 =		124.	142.67 ÷ 0.000 1 =
125.	3.0 ÷ 0.1 =		126.	89.06 ÷ 0.01 =
127.	111.2 ÷ 0.001 =		128.	0.001 02 ÷ 0.000 1 =
129.	175.01 ÷ 0.1 =		130.	13.031 ÷ 0.01 =

PERCENTAGES

The term *percent* means hundredths and is written as %. It is another way of stating a fraction. The number stated in a percentage is the numerator, and the denominator is always 100.

> *EXAMPLES:* 10% = 10/100
>
> ---
>
> $1/4\% = \dfrac{1/4}{100}$

To CONVERT a PERCENTAGE to a COMMON FRACTION:

A. Remove the percent sign and express as hundredths.

B. Write the given number as the numerator.

C. Write 100 as the denominator.

D. Reduce to lowest terms.

EXAMPLES: $10\% = {}^{10}/_{100} = {}^1/_{10}$

$${}^1/_4\% = \frac{1/4}{100} = {}^1/_4 \div 100 = {}^1/_4 \times {}^1/_{100} = {}^1/_{400}$$

$$15\,{}^1/_3\% = \frac{46/3}{100} = {}^{46}/_3 \div 100 = {}^{46}/_3 \times {}^1/_{100} =$$
$${}^{46}/_{300} = {}^{23}/_{150}$$

Convert the following percentages to common fractions:

131. ${}^1/_2\% =$ 132. $15\% =$

133. $28\% =$ 134. $3\,{}^1/_4\% =$

135. $53\% =$

To CONVERT a PERCENTAGE to a DECIMAL NUMBER:

A. Remove the percent sign.

B. Move the decimal two places to the left or divide by 100.

C. Add zeroes as required.

EXAMPLES: $50\% = 0.50$

$2\% = 0.02$

${}^1/_8\% = 0.125\% = 0.001\,25$

Convert the following percentages to decimal numbers:

136. $18\% =$ 137. $90\% =$

138. $7\,{}^1/_2\% =$ 139. $72\% =$

140. $8\% =$

To CONVERT a FRACTION to a PERCENTAGE:

A. Multiply the fraction by 100.

B. Divide the numerator by the denominator.

C. Add the percent sign (%).

D. Do not round off decimal numbers.

> EXAMPLES: $3/5 =$
> $$3/5 \times 100 =$$
> $$300/5 = 60 = 60\%$$
>
> _____
>
> $2/9 =$
> $$2/9 \times 100 =$$
> $$200/9 = 22.2 = 22.2\%$$

Convert the following fractions to percentages:

141.	$1/7 =$	142.	$3/11 =$
143.	$7 1/2 =$	144.	$1 2/5 =$
145.	$3/4 =$		

To CONVERT a DECIMAL NUMBER to a PERCENTAGE:

A. Move the decimal two places to the right or multiply by 100.

B. Add zeroes if required.

C. Add the percent sign.

> EXAMPLES: 0.6
> $$0.6 \times 100 = 60$$
> $$60 = 60\%$$

Convert the following decimal numbers to percentages:

146.   0.32 =   147.   0.101 6 =

148.   0.007 =   149.   1.001 5 =

150.   16.04 =

RATIOS

A *ratio* indicates a relationship between two numbers. It expresses a fraction. The two numbers are separated by a colon, which indicates division. When reading a ratio, the colon represents "is to."

> EXAMPLE: $1/2 = 1:2$
>
> Reads: one is to two.

To CONVERT a PROPER FRACTION to a RATIO:

A.   Reduce the fraction to lowest terms.

B.   Write the numerator to the left of the colon.

C.   Write the denominator to the right of the colon.

> EXAMPLE: $6/8 = 3/4 = 3:4$

Reduce the following proper fractions to lowest terms and convert to ratios:

151. $1/8$ =   152. $11/12$ =

153. $21/42$ =   154. $9/17$ =

155. $25/125$ =

To CONVERT a DECIMAL NUMBER to a RATIO:

A.   Convert the decimal number to a proper fraction.

B.   Reduce the fraction to lowest terms.

C. Write the numerator to the left of the colon.

D. Write the denominator to the right of the colon.

EXAMPLES: $0.25 = {}^{25}/100 = {}^{1}/4 = 1:4$

$0.35 = {}^{35}/100 = {}^{7}/20 = 7:20$

Convert the following decimal numbers to ratios and reduce to lowest terms:

156. 0.1 =   157. 0.215 =

158. 0.160 3 =   159. 0.794 2 =

160. 0.005 2 =

To CONVERT a RATIO to a FRACTION:

A. Write the number to the left of the colon as the numerator.

B. Write the number to the right of the colon as the denominator.

C. Reduce to lowest terms.

EXAMPLE: $10:16 = {}^{10}/16 = {}^{5}/8$

Convert the following ratios to fractions and reduce to lowest terms:

161. 3 : 15 =   162. 16 : 39 =

163. 14 : 53 =   164. 10 : 101 =

165. 7 : 13 =

To CONVERT a RATIO to a DECIMAL NUMBER:

A. Convert the ratio to a fraction.

B. Divide the numerator by the denominator.

EXAMPLE: $3:4 = {}^{3}/4 = 3 \div 4 = 0.75$

Convert the following ratios to decimal numbers:

166. $5:7 =$ 167. $10:50 =$

168. $12:31 =$ 169. $18:41 =$

170. $1:17 =$

To CONVERT a PERCENTAGE to a RATIO:

A.   Express the percentage as a fraction.

B.   Express the fraction as a ratio.

C.   Reduce to lowest terms.

EXAMPLE: $35\% = {}^{35}/_{100} = 35:100 = 7:20$

Convert the following percentages to ratios and reduce to lowest terms:

171. $12\% =$ 172. $60\% =$

173. $73\% =$ 174. $17\% =$

175. $8\% =$

To CONVERT a RATIO to a PERCENTAGE:

A.   Convert the ratio to a fraction.

B.   Multiply by 100.

C.   Divide the numerator by the denominator.

D.   Add the percent sign.

EXAMPLE: $4:5 = {}^{4}/_{5} \times 100 = {}^{400}/_{5} = 80 = 80\%$

Convert the following ratios to percentages:

176. $1:8 =$ 177. $3:7 =$

178. $11:24 =$ 179. $8:36 =$

180. $16:47 =$

PROPORTIONS

A proportion consists of two ratios of equal value. Their relationship is shown through the use of a double colon. When reading a proportion, the double colon represents "as."

> *EXAMPLE:*   1 : 2 :: 3 : 6
>
> Reads: One is to two as three is to six.

The first and fourth terms of a proportion are known as the *extremes.*

The second and third terms of a proportion are known as the *means.*

> *EXAMPLE:*   1 : 2 :: 3 : 6
>
> 1 and 6 are the extremes.
>
> 2 and 3 are the means.

Because the ratios are of equal value, the product of the means will equal the product of the extremes.

> *EXAMPLE:*   Product of means = Product of extremes
>
> 1 : 2 :: 3 : 6
>
> 2 x 3 = 1 x 6
>
> 6 = 6

Because the product of the means is known to equal the product of the extremes, any single unknown term in a proportion can be calculated. This unknown term is generally referred to as "X."

To CALCULATE the value of X:

A. Multiply the means.

B. Multiply the extremes.

C. Place the value with the X on the left.

D. Place the known value on the right.

E. Divide the terms of the entire equation by the number preceding X.

   EXAMPLE: $3:4::X:8$

   $4 \times X = 3 \times 8$

   $4X = 24$

   $X = {}^{24}/_4$

   $X = 6$

AN IMPORTANT POINT TO REMEMBER:

To CHECK CALCULATIONS when using a PROPORTION to solve unknown terms:

A. Replace X by the answer obtained.

B. Multiply the means.

C. Multiply the extremes.

D. Ensure that the means equal the extremes.

E. If the answers are not equal, an error in calculation has been made; **review proportion and all calculations.**

   EXAMPLE: $2:3::X:9$

   $3 \times X = 2 \times 9$

   $3X = 18$

   $X = {}^{18}/_3$

   $X = 6$

   Means $3 \times 6 = 18$

   Extremes $2 \times 9 = 18$

   Means (18) = (18) Extremes

Calculate the value of X:

181. $50:X::75:3 =$ 182. $3:4::20:X =$

183. $12:24::X:16 =$ 184. $X:6::9:18 =$

185. $9 : X :: 3 : 20 =$

186. $31 : 51 :: X : 100 =$

187. $X : 50 :: 5 : 60 =$

188. $300\ 000 : X :: 1\ 200\ 000 : 4 =$

189. $3/4 : 12 :: 4 : X =$

190. $1/3 : X :: 4/5 : 7 =$

191. $1/2 : X :: 2/3 : 1/5 =$

192. $X : 1/5 :: 2 : 3 =$

193. $X : 1/2 :: 5 : 8 =$

194. $1/10 : 5 :: 10 : X =$

195. $0.9 : 6 :: X : 4 =$

196. $2.6 : X :: 3.9 : 0.5 =$

197. $X : 0.11 :: 1.0 : 0.1 =$

198. $0.75 : 3 :: 0.5 : X =$

199. $0.4 : 8 :: 1.6 : X =$

200. $0.15 : 2 :: 0.3 : X =$

CHAPTER 3:
METRIC SYSTEM

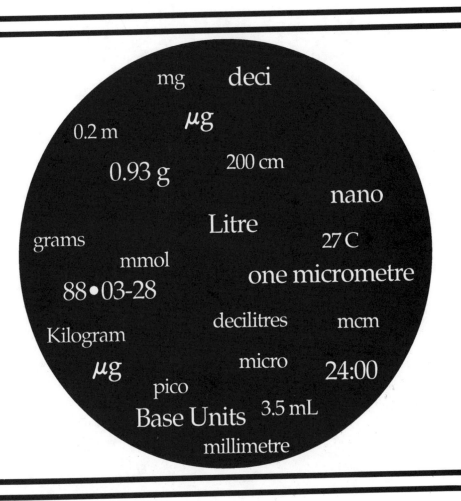

CHAPTER 3

Objectives

1. The student will demonstrate an understanding of the metric system as it applies to health care.

2. The student will demonstrate the ability to solve metric system equivalents accurately.

3. The student will demonstrate the ability to write symbols and numbers in the metric system.

4. The student will demonstrate the ability to speak and write 24-hour time.

5. The student will demonstrate the ability to write dates in the metric system.

WHY CHANGE TO METRIC?

The *apothecary* and *household* systems of measurement present problems with calculations because neither has a base unit. Their origins are varied, and therefore no definite standards apply. Over the years, local adaptations have added alternate and varied equivalencies. Although North America originally adopted these traditional systems of measurement, there is a definite movement towards the metric system.

The metric system stems back to France, approximately 200 years ago. Since then, various versions have been developed. The metric system has a base unit of 10, which applies to all areas of measurement. It has proved to be so effective that it has been adopted by 98% of the world's population.[1]

Despite conversion to the metric system, physicians may still order certain drugs using the apothecary or household systems, for example "1 teaspoon of cough syrup." See Appendix O for common conversions between the systems of measurement.

The current metric system that has replaced all former metric and non-metric systems of measurement is the SI system. This comes from the French name, le Système international d'unités. SI is founded on seven *"base units."* Any physical quantity can be expressed in SI using combinations of these base units.

Base Units

Three base units relevant to dosage calculation are found in Figure 3-1. See Appendix L for the remaining base units.

---

[1] SI Manual in Health Care, 2nd Ed. 1982 10.06, p.1.

QUANTITY	BASE UNIT	SI SYMBOL
Length	metre	m
Mass*	kilogram	kg
Amount of substance	mole	mol

* The gram (g) will replace kilogram (kg) as the base unit for calculating mass, to eliminate confusion with prefixes.

Figure 3-1:   SI base units relevant to dosage calculation.

The SI unit for volume is the cubic metre; however, the litre is the recommended unit of volume for fluids. Concentrations of solutions are expressed in litres (L) or its subunits.

Prefixes

The entire metric system is derived by combining the base units with standard prefixes used in the system. These prefixes are derived from multiples of 10. Figure 3-2 lists the prefixes relevant to health care and their appropriate symbols and values. The use of these prefixes converts a base unit to a subunit.

PREFIX	SYMBOL	VALUE
kilo	k	1 000 times a base unit
deci	d	0.1 (one tenth) of a base unit
centi	c	0.01 (one hundredth) of a base unit
milli	m	0.001 (one thousandth) of a base unit
micro	μ or mc	0.000 001 (one millionth) of a base unit
nano	n	0.000 000 001 (one billionth) of a base unit
pico	p	0.000 000 000 001 (one trillionth) of a base unit

Figure 3-2: Metric prefixes relevant to health care.

NOTE: See Appendix C for answers to questions in this chapter.

Complete the following statements:

1. The metric system is replacing the _____ and _____ systems of measurement.

2. SI is founded on seven units called _____.

3. The metric system has a base unit of _____.

4. The _____ is the recommended unit for measuring volume of fluids.

5. The metric prefix _____ indicates 1 000 times a base unit.

Give abbreviations for the following:

6.   gram   _____

7.   millilitre   _____

8.   litre   _____

9.   milligram _____

10. kilogram   _____

11. nanomole _____

12. centimetre _____

13. metre   _____

14. kilo   _____

15. milli   _____

Conversions

To CONVERT a BASE UNIT or SUBUNIT:

A.   Use fractions or multiples of 10 as indicated.

EXAMPLE: Centi = 0.01 (one hundredth) of a base unit

1 cm = 0.01 ($^1/_{100}$) m

One hundred centimetres equals one metre, therefore, 100 cm = 1 m.

To CONVERT a LARGER unit to a SMALLER unit:

A.   Multiply or move the decimal to the right. Other known ratios may also be used in a proportion to solve for X.

EXAMPLES: Convert 2 m to cm

METHOD #1: 2 m = X cm

centi = 0.01 of a base unit

1 cm = 0.01 m

X cm = 2 m

1 cm : 0.01 m : : X cm : 2 m

$$0.01 \text{ m } \times \text{ X cm } = 1 \text{ cm } \times 2 \text{ m}$$

$$0.01 \text{ X } = 2$$

$$\text{X } = {}^2/_{0.01}$$

$$\text{X } = 200$$

$$2 \text{ m } = 200 \text{ cm}$$

METHOD #2:   m = X cm

cm = 0.01, which is two decimal places

Move the decimal in 2 m two places to the

right.

2.0 m = 200.0 cm

METHOD #3:   1 m = 100 cm
2 m =   X cm

1 m : 100 cm : : 2 m : X cm

1 m × X cm = 100 cm × 2 m

1X = 200

$$\text{X } = {}^{200}/_1$$

X = 200 cm

NOTE: Although this text solves for X using proportions, an alternate method can be used. This method cross-multiplies the equivalent terms, resulting in the same equivalency as multiplying the means and the extremes. The step of setting up the proportion is eliminated.

EXAMPLE: 1 m = 100 cm
2 m = X cm

1 m × X cm = 2 m × 100 cm

1 X = 200

$$\text{X } = {}^{200}/_1$$

X = 200 cm

Convert the following larger units to smaller units:

16. 3 kg = _____ g

17. 0.25 L = _____ mL

18. 0.10 L = _____ mL

19. 5.3 g = _____ mg

20. 0.1 g = _____ mcg

21. 0.75 g = _____ mg

22. 10 mg = _____ µg

23. 2 kg = _____ mcg

24. 1 kg = _____ mg

25. 5 mol = _____ mmol

26. 0.30 kg =_____ g

27. 1.8 kg = _____ g

28. 0.95 L = _____ mL

29. 300 g = _____ mg

30. 7 cm = _____ mm

31. 2.1 L = _____ mL

32. 15 g = _____ mg

33. 1.9 kg = _____ g

34. 8.5 L = _____ mL

35. 2.3 L = _____ mL

36. 5.1 L = _____ mL

37. 90 g = _____ mg

38. 115 g = _____ mg

39. 7.5 m = _____ mm

40. 3.2 mol =_____ mmol

41. 0.85 kg =_____ mg

42. 12 cm = _____ mcm

43. 8 mol = _____ mmol

44. 3 kg = _____ mg

45. 10 L = _____ dL

46.　1.1 L = _____ mL

47.　0.25 dL = _____ mL

48.　15 cm = _____ mm

49.　1.5 m = _____ cm

50.　1.5 m = _____ mm

To CONVERT a SMALLER unit to a LARGER unit:

A. Divide or move the decimal to the left. Other known ratios may also be used in a proportion to solve for X.

EXAMPLES: Convert 3 mm to m

METHOD#1: 3 mm = X m

milli = 0.001 of a base unit

1 mm = 0.001 m
3 mm = X m

1 mm : 0.001 m : : 3 mm : X m

1 mm x X m = 0.001 m x 3 mm

1 X = 0.003

$X = {0.003}/1$

X = 0.003

3 mm = 0.003 m

METHOD #2: 3 mm = X m

mm = 0.001, which is three decimal places.
Move the decimal in 3 m three places to the left.

3.0 mm = 0.003 m

METHOD #3: 1 000 mm = 1 m
3 mm = X m

1 000 mm : 1 m : : 3 mm : X m

1 000 mm x X m = 1 m x 3 mm

1 000 X = 3

$$X = {}^3/_{1\,000}$$
$$X = 0.003 \text{ m}$$

Convert the following smaller units to larger units:

51.   400 mg = _____ g

52.   610 mL = _____ L

53.   1 010 mg = _____ g

54.   90 mcg = _____ mg

55.   450 g = _____ kg

56.   95 mL = _____ L

57.   5 000 mg = _____ g

58.   250 mL = _____ L

59.   115 mL = _____ L

60.   3 650 dL = _____ L

61.   1 520 g = _____ kg

62.   68 mL = _____ dL

63.   158 mL = _____ dL

64.   450 mL = _____ L

65.   2 350 mL = _____ L

66.   325 mg = _____ g

67.   4 mm = _____ cm

68.   16 mmol = _____ mol

69.   25 mmol = _____ mol

70.   0.5 mmol = _____ mol

71.   5 dL = _____ L

72.   1 500 g = _____ kg

73.   0.05 mcg = _____ mg

74.   2 500 mL = _____ L

75.   500 μg = _____ kg

76.   360 mg = _____ kg

77.   1 050 mg = _____ kg

78.   116 cm = _____ m

79.   0.9 mcm = _____ cm

80.   0.75 μm = _____ mm

81.   100 mm = _____ cm

82.   45 mm = _____ cm

83.   306 μm = _____ m

84.   97 cm = _____ m

85.   2.1 mm = _____ m

Base Units

The following is a summary of the base units applicable to health care. Prefixes relevant to each unit are listed with equivalents. Appropriate symbols are given. Familiarity with these equivalents will facilitate working with the metric system.

LENGTH: Base unit   = metre (m)*

= 10 decimetres (dm)

= 100 centimetres (cm)

1 metre (m)   = 1 000 millimetres (mm)

= 1 000 000 micrometres (μm or mcm)

= 0.001 kilometre (km)

Figure 3-3 shows the actual relationship of millimetres to centimetres.

---

* This text will use metre, although meter is also acceptable.

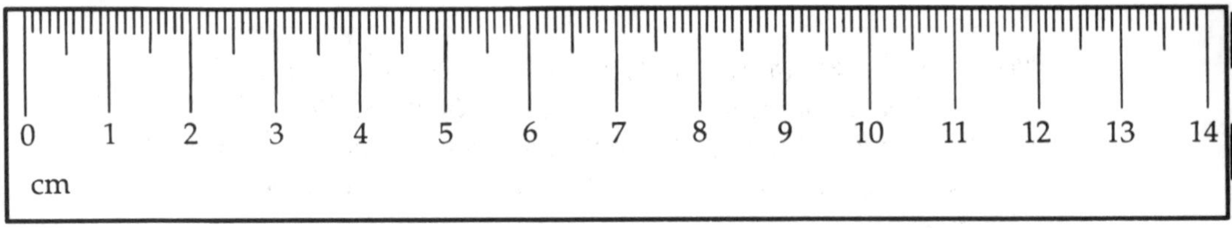

Figure 3-3 : A metric ruler.

MASS: Base unit   = gram (g)

1 gram (g)   {
= 1 000 milligrams (mg)
= 1 000 000 micrograms (μg or mcg)
= 0.001 kilogram (kg)

AMOUNT OF SUBSTANCE: Base unit = mole (mol)

1 mole (mol) {
= 1 000 millimoles (mmol)
= 1 000 000 micromoles (μmol or mcmol)
= 1 000 000 000 nanomoles (nmol)
= 1 000 000 000 000 picomoles (pmol)

VOLUME: Base unit   = litre (L)*

1 litre (L) {
= 1 000 millilitres (mL)

= 10 decilitres (dL)

In keeping with SI recommendations, cubic centimetre (cc) is to be replaced by millilitre (mL) to express fluid volume.

---

* This text will use litre, although liter is also acceptable.

THE DEGREE CELSIUS

The unit of temperature is the degree Celsius (°C). It is the accepted measurement of temperature because the Kelvin scale has limited application in medicine; it begins at absolute zero (-273°C). Figure 3-4 shows the Celsius scale on a clinical thermometer.

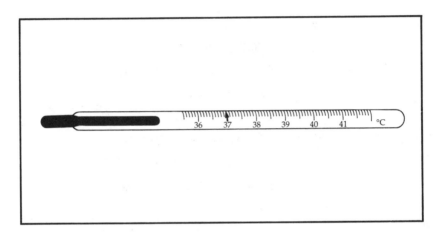

Figure 3-4:   A Celsius thermometer.

To WRITE SYMBOLS in the METRIC SYSTEM:

A.   Use lower-case letters unless the name of the unit comes from a proper name.
The symbol is then written in upper case.

EXAMPLES: gram = g

_____

newton = N

The only other unit that deviates from this rule is the litre, written as L, to avoid confusion with the number 1.

B. Never pluralize symbols.

EXAMPLES: 15 g NOT gs

_____

1 200 mL NOT 1 200 mLs

C. Never use a period except at the end of a sentence.

EXAMPLES: 25 cm NOT 25 cm.

_____

2.5 mg NOT 2.5 mg.

D. Use a full space between a number and symbol unless the first character of a symbol is not a letter. The number and symbol are then written without a space.

EXAMPLES: 12 mm NOT 12mm

_____

24°C NOT 24 °C

To WRITE NUMBERS in the METRIC SYSTEM:

A. Never mix words and symbols.

EXAMPLES: 10 mL NOT ten mL

_____

3 g NOT three g

B. Use decimals, not fractions.

EXAMPLES: 0.50 g NOT $^1/_2$ g

_____

0.25 mL NOT $^1/_4$ mL

C. It is recommended that a long number be spaced into three-digit sections to facilitate reading. This space replaces the traditional comma.

EXAMPLES: 19 678 352.107 321, NOT 19678352.107321

---

1 000 mL NOT 1,000 mL

D. Always place a zero before the decimal when the number is less than one.

EXAMPLES: 0.10 mg NOT .10 mg

0.5 L NOT .5 L

Read the following measurements carefully and state whether they are correct or incorrect. If they are incorrect, state the correct answer:

86.   15g
87.   96 gs
88.   .6 L
89.   0.49 G
90.   Six millilitres
91.   10 °C
92.   thirty g
93.   8 cm
94.   1 g.
95.   1,000 mL
96.   43 kg
97. $^1/_2$ mmol
98.   2.3 1
99.   7 μgs
100.   19 mol

24-HOUR TIME

The 24-hour clock expresses time as four digits commencing at midnight with 00:00 or 24:00. The first two digits express the number of hours since midnight; the last two digits express the number of minutes in that hour.

It is important to note that second(s) is the only SI unit of time. The 24-hour clock is included in this chapter because it is widely used in the health care system.

To WRITE 24-hour time:

A.   Time is always expressed with a minimum of four digits.

B.   The first two digits indicate the number of hours past midnight. If the hour is less than 10, the first digit will be zero.

EXAMPLES: 7 a.m. = 07:00

_____

7 p.m. = 19:00

C.   The second two digits indicate the number of minutes past the hour. If less than 10 minutes have passed, the first digit will be zero.

EXAMPLES: 7:09 a.m. = 07:09

_____

7:09 p.m. = 19:09

D.   Each pair of digits is separated by a colon.

E.   When writing time, the terms *hours* or *minutes* are not used.

F.   To write seconds, a colon and two more digits are added to the right of the time.

EXAMPLES: 04:30:21

_____

15:03:09

To SPEAK 24-hour time:

A.   Each pair of digits is expressed as a separate whole number. Zeroes are expressed individually.

   EXAMPLES: 00:19 is expressed as zero-zero nineteen.

   _____

   06:45 is expressed as zero-six forty-five.

   _____

   11:05 is expressed as eleven zero-five.

   _____

   15:27 is expressed as fifteen twenty-seven.

B.   When reading time, the terms *hours* or *minutes* are not expressed.

To CALCULATE 24-hour time:

NOTE: Midnight is time point zero (00:00 or 24:00).

A.   12:00 a.m. (midnight) to 12:59 a.m.

   00:00 to 00:59   Here no hours have passed from midnight
        or   to 1:00 a.m.; therefore, only minutes are
   24:00 to 00:59   expressed in the four-digit format.

           EXAMPLES: 12:34 a.m. = 00:34

           _____

           12:57 a.m. = 00:57

B: 1:00 a.m. to 12:00 p.m. (noon)

   01:00 to 12:00   Here all hours and minutes are expressed in
                    the four-digit format.

           EXAMPLES: 9:15 a.m. = 09:15

           _____

           10:47 a.m. = 10:47

C.   12:01 p.m. to 12:00 a.m.(midnight)

12:01 to 24:00   Here 12:00 is added to all expressions
       or   of time, resulting in the four-digit
12:01 to 00:0   format.

> *EXAMPLES:*   2:38 p.m. =
>   2:38 + 12:00 =
>   14:38
>   _____
>
>   10:47 p.m. =
>   10:47 + 12:00 =
>   22:47

Figure 3-5 shows how to calculate 24-hour time.

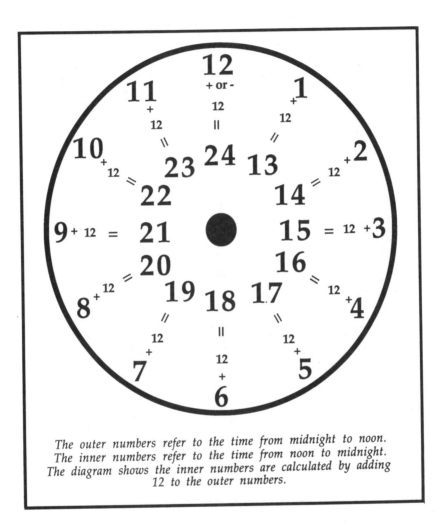

The outer numbers refer to the time from midnight to noon.
The inner numbers refer to the time from noon to midnight.
The diagram shows the inner numbers are calculated by adding
12 to the outer numbers.

Figure 3-5: Calculating 24-hour time.

Convert the following traditional times to their 24-hour equivalent:

101.	7:35 a.m.	102.	12:00 noon
103.	10:23 a.m.	104.	5:30 p.m.
105.	11:00 p.m.	106.	2 53 a.m.
107.	7:35 p.m.	108.	12:00 midnight
109.	12:05 a.m.	110.	9:17 p.m.

THE DATE IN METRIC

To WRITE the DATE in metric:

A. The sequence is year, month, and day.

   EXAMPLE: December 22, 1987 = 87•12•22

B. Each category is always expressed by two digits. If the month or day is less than 10, the first digit will be zero.

   EXAMPLES: January 9, 1988 = 88•01•09

   February 14, 1990 = 90•02•14

C. A consistent marker, such as a dot or dash, separates the three categories.

   EXAMPLES: February 24, 1988 = 88•02•24

   March 1, 1988 = 88-03-01

Write the following dates in metric:

111.	January 1, 1989	112.	July 3, 1982
113.	July 8, 1977	114.	March 28, 1985
115.	September 9, 1954		

CHAPTER 4:
ORAL DOSAGES

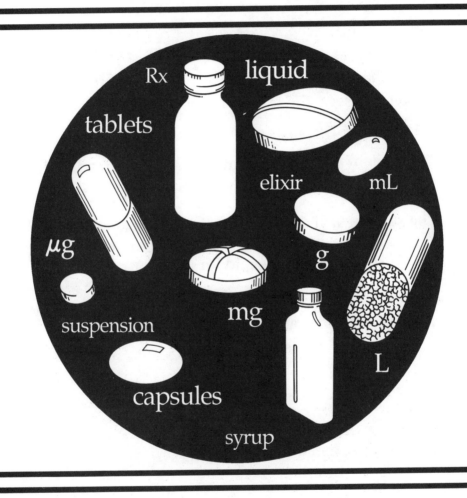

CHAPTER 4

Objectives

1. The student will demonstrate an understanding of the term *dosage*, the factors influencing it and relevant terms.

2. The student will demonstrate the ability to read and understand a physician's medication order.

3. The student will demonstrate the ability to calculate accurately the amount of oral medication to administer for one dose and for a 24-hour period.

4. The student will demonstrate the ability to calculate a child's dose of oral medication accurately.

DOSAGES

The term *dosage* refers to the determination and control of the size and number of dosages.

A *dose* is the amount of medication administered at a specific time.

DOSE LEVELS

A *minimal dose* is the smallest dose that produces a therapeutic effect.

A *maximal dose* is the largest dose that can be administered without causing undesirable results.

A *therapeutic range* is the range of doses, between the minimal and maximal dose, that produces a desired effect.

A *toxic dose* is a dose that results in a poisonous effect. This may occur from an initial toxic dose or from a cumulative effect, after repeated administration of a medication.

A *lethal dose* is a dose that is large enough to result in death.

A number of factors influence the dosage of medication administered to an individual. A summary of these factors follows.

FACTORS THAT INFLUENCE DOSAGE:

AGE: Children and older adults generally require smaller dosages than young to middle-aged adults.

BODY SIZE: Small-framed or underweight individuals may require smaller dosages, and likewise, large-framed or overweight individuals may require larger dosages.

PHYSICAL CONDITION: The physical condition of an individual is a grave consideration in the administration and evaluation of medications. Smaller dosages may be required when an underlying medical condition potentiates the action of a medication. An individual in pain may require larger dosages.

EMOTIONAL: The emotional state of an individual may require alterations in recommended dosages.

ROUTE: The route of administration may influence the dosage. Some medications administered orally require larger dosages than the same medications administered parenterally.

ABSORPTION AND EXCRETION: The rate of absorption and excretion in an individual's system may affect dosage. If absorption is fast and excretion slow, dosages may be decreased to avoid toxicity.

ORDERS

A physician writes an *order* for the preparation and administration of medications. The order may be written using abbreviations. Each order (Figure 4-1) should contain the following information, not necessarily in this sequence:

A. Generic or trade name of medication.

B. Dose to be administered.

C. Route of administration.

D. Frequency of administration.

E. Reason for administration.

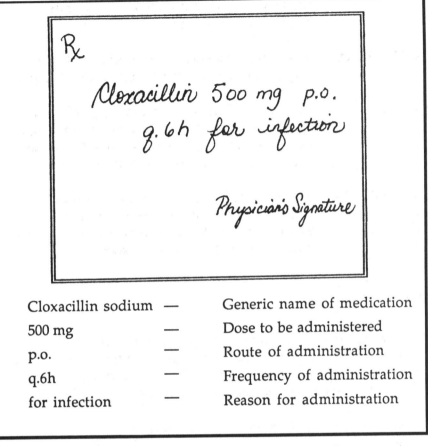

Cloxacillin sodium	—	Generic name of medication
500 mg	—	Dose to be administered
p.o.	—	Route of administration
q.6h	—	Frequency of administration
for infection	—	Reason for administration

Figure 4-1: Components of a medication order.

The following information is necessary for the safe preparation and administration of medications:

A. The maximal and minimal doses of the medication.

B. The actions, indications, and adverse effects of the medication.

C. The abbreviations and symbols relevant to medication administration. See Appendix K for common abbreviations and symbols.

It is *crucial* that all doses be *calculated correctly.*

ORAL DOSAGES

The oral route is the preferred method for administration of medications.

Advantages

A.   Administration is convenient, because the route is accessible, comfortable, and preferred by most individuals.

B.   The skin is not broken; therefore, there is less risk of infection.

C.   Production costs are lower than other routes; therefore, it is more economical.

Disadvantages

A.   The alimentary canal may be irritated.

B.   Calculation of accurate dosages is difficult because absorption occurs mainly in the small intestine.

C.   Administration is difficult, or impossible, when an individual is irrational or unconscious.

D.   Administration is contraindicated if an individual is N.P.O.

The most common oral medications are tablets, capsules, and liquids. Scored tablets have indentations allowing for easy division when only part of the medication is to be administered. See Figure 4-2 for examples of various oral medications.

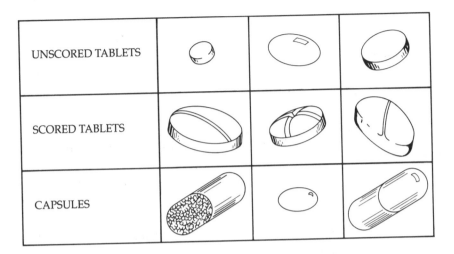

UNSCORED TABLETS			
SCORED TABLETS			
CAPSULES			

Figure 4-2: Various oral medications.

To CALCULATE ORAL DOSES from TABLETS and CAPSULES:

Calculation of the amount of medication to be administered orally may be required if:

A. The amount of the medication available is different from what is ordered. For example, the physician orders 500 mg and only 250-mg tablets are available.

B. The dose of the medication is ordered, but the amount required to provide this dose is not specified. For example, the physician orders 2 g of a medication, available in capsules, but does not specify the number of capsules.

Calculation of the number of tablets or capsules to be administered is required in these situations.

A general formula (Figure 4-3) for calculating the amount of medication to be administered can be used to calculate the number of tablets or capsules required for each dose of an oral medication.

$$\frac{\text{DOSE DESIRED}}{\text{DOSE ON HAND}} \times \text{DRUG FORM} = \text{AMOUNT TO ADMINISTER}$$

The *dose desired* is the dose of medication to be administered.
The *dose on hand* is the dose of medication available.
The *drug form* is how the medication is supplied. It is equivalent to the dose on hand.

Figure 4-3: General formula for calculating medications.

NOTE: When using the above formula, remember:

A.   The dose desired and the dose on hand must be expressed in like terms.

B.   The drug form is always equivalent to the dose on hand.

C.   Recheck your calculations if the amount to administer is unrealistic.

D.   The words *drug* and *medication* are interchangeable.

An alternate method for calculating the number of tablets or capsules uses ratios.

EXAMPLE #1: The physician's order reads:

Lanoxin 0.0625 mg   p.o. o.d.

Digoxin (Lanoxin) is available in 0.125-mg tablets. How many tablets will be administered for each dose?

METHOD #1

$$\frac{\text{Dose Desired}}{\text{Dose on Hand}} \times \text{Drug Form} = \text{Amount to Administer}$$

$$\frac{0.062\,5 \text{ mg}}{0.125 \text{ mg}} \times 1 \text{ tab.} =$$

$$0.125\,\overline{)0.062\,5} = 125\,\overline{)62.5}^{.5} = 0.5$$

0.5 x 1 tab. = 0.5 tab.

METHOD #2

0.125 mg = 1 tab.
0.062 5 mg = X tab.

0.125 mg : 1 tab. : : 0.062 5 mg : X tab.

0.125 x X = 1 x 0.062 5

0.125X = 0.062 5

X = 0.062 5/0.125

X = 0.5 tab.

There will be 0.5 tab. administered for each dose.

NOTE: Throughout this text, when two medication names are given, the generic name is followed by a trade name in parentheses.

EXAMPLE #2: The physician's order reads:

magnesium gluconate 1.5 g p.o. o.d.

Magnesium gluconate (Maglucate) is available in 500-mg tablets. How many tablets will be administered for each dose?

NOTE: The dose desired is in grams and the dose on hand is in milligrams. The first step in this problem is to change grams to milligrams.

1 g   = 1 000 mg
1.5 g = X mg

Set up a ratio

1 g : 1 000 mg : : 1.5 g : X mg

1 x X = 1 000 x 1.5

$$1X = 1\,500$$
$$X = {}^{1\,500}/_1$$
$$X = 1\,500 \text{ mg}$$

Or

Move the decimal three places to the right.

$$1.5 = 1\,500 \text{ mg}$$

METHOD #1

$$\frac{\text{Dose Desired}}{\text{Dose on Hand}} \times \text{Drug Form} = \text{Amount to Administer}$$

$$\frac{1\,500 \text{ mg}}{500 \text{ mg}} \times 1 \text{ tab.} =$$

$$500 \overline{)\,1\,500\,} = 3 \quad \overset{3}{}$$

$$3 \times 1 \text{ tab.} = 3 \text{ tabs.}$$

METHOD #2

$$500 \text{ mg} = 1 \text{ tab.}$$
$$1\,500 \text{ mg} = X \text{ tab.}$$

$$500 \text{ mg} : 1 \text{ tab.} : : 1\,500 \text{ mg} : X \text{ tab.}$$

$$500 \times X = 1 \times 1\,500$$

$$500X = 1\,500$$

$$X = {}^{1\,500}/_{500}$$

$$X = 3 \text{ tabs.}$$

There will be 3 tabs. administered for each dose.

NOTE: No one method must be used exclusively. Varying methods may be used effectively to obtain the same answer. In Example #2, the formula for calculating oral medications, the ratio method, and the metric method for converting a larger to a smaller unit were used.

EXAMPLE #3: The physician's order reads:

Vasotec 2.5 mg p.o. o.d.

Enalapril (Vasotec) is available in 5-mg tablets scored in half. How many tablets will be administered for each dose? How many tablets will be administered in a 24-hour period?

METHOD #1

$$\frac{\text{Dose Desired}}{\text{Dose on Hand}} \times \text{Drug Form} = \text{Amount to Administer}$$

$$\frac{2.5 \text{ mg}}{5 \text{ mg}} \times 1 \text{ tab.} =$$

$$5\overline{)2.5}^{\,0.5} = 0.5$$

0.5 x 1 tab. = 0.5 tab.

There will be 0.5 tab. administered for each dose.

To CALCULATE the AMOUNT to ADMINISTER in a 24-HOUR PERIOD:

A. Identify the frequency of administration and determine the number of doses to be administered in a 24-hour period. It is important to know abbreviations. See Appendix K.

B. Determine the amount to administer for each dose and multiply this by the number of doses in a 24-hour period.

EXAMPLE: o.d. = once a day = the frequency of administration

0.5 tab. = the amount to administer for each dose

0.5 x 1 = 0.5 tab.

0.5 tab. will be administered in a 24-hour period.

EXAMPLE #4: The physician's order reads:

Cloxacillin sodium 0.5 g p.o. q.6h

Cloxacillin sodium (Orbenin) is available in 250-mg capsules. How many capsules will be administered for each dose?

First convert

0.5 g to mg

1 g = 1 000 mg
0.5 g = X mg

1 g : 1 000 mg : : 0.5 g : X mg

1 x X = 1 000 x 0.5

1 X = 500

X = $500/1$

X = 500 mg

Or

Move the decimal three places to the right.

0.5 g = 500 mg

METHOD #2

250 mg = 1 cap.
500 mg = X cap.

250 mg : 1 cap. : : 500 mg : X cap.

250 x X = 1 x 500

250X = 500

X = $500/250$

X = 2

There will be 2 caps. administered for each dose.

NOTE: See Appendix D for answers to questions in this
             chapter.

Calculate the number of tablets or capsules administered for
each dose and for a 24-hour period:

1.   Methyldopa (Aldomet) 500 mg p.o. b.i.d. The medication is
      available in 250-mg tablets.

2.   Hydralazine (Apresoline) 50 mg p.o. q.i.d. The medication
      is available in 50-mg tablets.

3.   Clomipramine (Anafranil) 200 mg p.o. h.s. The medication
      is available in 25-mg tablets.

4.   Captopril (Capoten) 6.25 mg p.o. t.i.d. The medication is
      available in 25-mg tablets scored in quarters.

5.   Senna glucosides (Glysennid) 17.2 mg p.o. h.s. The
      medication is available in 8.6-mg tablets.

6.   Benztropine mesylate (Cogentin) 1 mg p.o. h.s. The
      medication is available in 2-mg tablets scored in half.

7.   Erythromycin estolate (Ilosone) 0.5 g p.o. q.12h. The
      medication is available in 250-mg capsules.

8.   Theophylline (Somophyllin-12) 200 mg p.o. b.i.d. The
      medication is available in 100-mg capsules.

9.   Flurazepam HCl (Dalmane) 30 mg p.o. h.s. p.r.n. The
      medication is available in 15-mg capsules.

10. Alprazolam (Xanax) 0.25 mg p.o. t.i.d. and 1 mg h.s. The
      medication is available in 250-μg tablets.

To CALCULATE ORAL DOSES from LIQUID:

The previously stated formulae for calculating the amount
of medication to be administered are also used for liquids.

Medications in liquid form contain a given amount of drug
in a given amount of solution. Oral medications are generally
calculated in mL and poured into a graduated medicine cup.
(Figure 4-4).

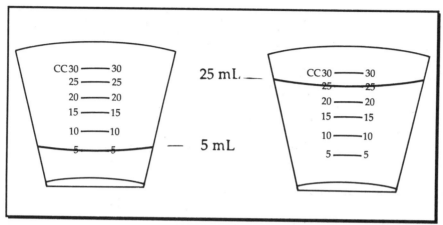

Figure 4-4: Graduated medicine cups.

EXAMPLE #1: The physician's order reads:

Gravol liquid 75 mg p.o. q.4h p.r.n.

Dimenhydrinate (Gravol) liquid is available in 15 mg per 5 mL. How many mL will be administered for each dose?

METHOD #1

$$\frac{\text{Dose Desired}}{\text{Dose on Hand}} \text{ x Drug Form } = \text{ Amount to Administer}$$

$$\frac{75 \text{ mg}}{15 \text{ mg}} \text{ x } 5 \text{ mL } =$$

AN IMPORTANT FACT TO REMEMBER: the drug form is NOT always 1.

$$15 \overline{)75} = 5$$

5 x 5 mL = 25 mL

METHOD #2

15 mg = 5 mL
75 mg = X mL

15 mg : 5 mL : : 75mg : XmL

15 x X = 5 x 75

15X = 375

$X = {}^{375}/_{15}$

X = 25 mL

There will be 25 mL administered for each dose.

EXAMPLE #2: The physician's order reads:

Benadryl elixir 50 mg p.o. t.i.d.

Diphenhydramine HCl (Benadryl) elixir is available in 12.5 mg per 5 mL. How many mL will be administered for each dose?

METHOD #1

$$\frac{\text{Dose Desired}}{\text{Dose on Hand}} \text{ x Drug Form } = \text{ Amount to Administer}$$

$$\frac{50 \text{ mg}}{12.5 \text{ mg}} \text{ x } 5 \text{ mL } =$$

$12.5\overline{)50} = 125\overline{)500} = 4$

4 x 5 mL = 20 mL

METHOD #2

12.5 mg = 5 mL
50 mg = X mL

12.5mg : 5 mL : : 50mg : XmL

12.5 x X = 5 x 50

12.5X = 250

$X = {}^{250}/_{12.5}$

X = 20 mL

There will be 20 mL administered for each dose.

EXAMPLE #3:   The physician's order reads:

Amoxil suspension 0.25g p.o. q.8h

Amoxicillin trihydrate (Amoxil) suspension is available in 125 mg per 5 mL. How many mL will be administered for each dose? How many mL will be administered in a 24-hour period?

First convert

0.25 g to mg

1 g = 1 000 mg
0.25 g = X mg

1 g : 1 000 mg : : 0.25 g : X mg

1 x X = 1 000 x 0.25

1X = 250

X = $^{250}/_1$

X = 250 mg

Or

Move the decimal three places to the right.

0.25 g = 250 mg

METHOD #1

$$\frac{\text{Dose Desired}}{\text{Dose on Hand}} \times \text{Drug Form} = \text{Amount to Administer}$$

$$\frac{250 \text{ mg}}{125 \text{ mg}} \times 5 \text{ mL} =$$

$$125 \overline{)\, 250} = 2$$

2 x 5 mL = 10 mL

There will be 10 mL administered for each dose.

q.8h = every 8 hours = 3 times in 24 hours

10 mL x 3 = 30 mL

30 mL will be administered in a 24-hour period.

EXAMPLE #4: The physician's order reads:

Docusate sodium syrup 100 mg p.o. b.i.d.

Docusate sodium (Colace) syrup is available in 20 mg per 5 mL. How many mL will be administered for each dose? How many mL will be administered in a 24-hour period?

METHOD #2

20 mg = 5 mL
100 mg = X mL

20 mg : 5 mL : : 100 mg : X mL

20 x X = 5 x 100

20X = 500

X = 500/20

X = 25

There will be 25 mL administered for each dose.

b.i.d. = twice a day = 2 times in 24 hours

25 mL x 2 = 50 mL

50 mL will be administered in a 24-hour period.

Calculate the amount of liquid administered for each dose and for a 24-hour period:

11. Acetaminophen (Tylenol) elixir 300 mg p.o. q.6h. The medication is available in 120 mg per 5 mL.

12. Dicloxacillin sodium monohydrate (Dynapen) suspension 125 mg p.o. q.i.d. The medication is available in 62.5 mg per mL.

13. Astemizole (Hismanal) suspension 5 mg p.o. o.d. The medication is available in 2 mg per mL.

14. Dicyclomine HCl (Bentylol) syrup 15 mg p.o. t.i.d. The medication is available in 10 mg per 5 mL.

15. Erythromycin estolate (Ilosone) liquid 0.5 g p.o. b.i.d. The medication is available in 250 mg per 5 mL.

16. Thioridazine HCl (Mellaril) suspension 25 mg p.o. t.i.d. The medication is available in 10 mg per 5 mL.

17. Oxtriphylline (Choledyl) elixir 250 mg p.o. q.i.d. The medication is available in 100 mg per 5 mL.

18. Aluminum hydroxide (Amphojel) liquid 640 mg p.o. q.4h. The medication is available in 320 mg per 5 mL.

19. Theophylline (Theolair) liquid 200 mg p.o. q.6h. The medication is available in 80 mg per 15 mL.

20. Docusate sodium (Colace) syrup 200 mg p.o. o.d. The medication is available in 4 mg per mL.

To CALCULATE ORAL DOSES for CHILDREN:

Dosages of medication administered to children are generally smaller than adult dosages. The amount administered is usually based on a fraction of the adult dosage. Body weight calculation is the most commonly used formula. This formula is metric and will be discussed in this chapter.

There are other formulae (rules) for calculating children's dosages (Appendix M).

These formulae do not always allow for the individual variations in body size, relevant to age. For example, using calculations requiring age only, an obese four-year-old could receive less than the minimal dose of medication. Conversely, a two-year-old of less than recommended weight could receive a toxic dose.

The *Compendium of Pharmaceuticals and Specialties* (CPS) lists the dosages of many medications for children in milligrams (mg) or micrograms (mcg or µg) per kilogram (kg) of weight.

A general formula (Figure 4-5) for calculating a child's dose can be used for oral medications.

DRUG DOSE X CHILD'S WEIGHT = CHILD'S DOSE
(in mg/kg)   (in kilograms)

Figure 4-5: Formula for a child's dose.

EXAMPLE: The CPS states that a child's dose of amoxicillin trihydrate (Amoxil) is 25 mg/kg administered in equally divided doses q.8h. Amoxicillin trihydrate pediatric drops are available in 50 mg per 1 mL. Calculate the dose for a child weighing 18 kg. How many mL will be administered for each dose?

DRUG DOSE x CHILD'S WEIGHT = CHILD'S DOSE
(in mg/kg)   (in kilograms)

---

25 mg/kg x 18 kg = 450 mg

Child's dose for a 24-hour period = 450 mg

450 mg in equal doses q.8h =

450 mg ÷ 3 = 150 mg

150 mg will be administered q.8h.

The child's dose can be used in the general formulae to calculate the amount of medication to administer.

METHOD #1

$$\frac{\text{Dose Desired}}{\text{Dose on Hand}} \times \text{Drug Form} = \text{Amount to Administer}$$

$$\frac{150 \text{ mg}}{50 \text{ mg}} \times 1 \text{ mL} =$$

$$50 \overline{)150} = 50 \overline{)150}^{\,3} = 3$$

$$3 \times 1 \text{ mL} = 3 \text{ mL}$$

METHOD #2

50 mg = 1 mL
150 mg = X mL

50 mg : 1 mL : : 150 mg : X mL

50 x X = 1 x 150

50X = 150

X = $^{150}/_{50}$

X = 3 mL

There will be 3 mL administered for each dose.

Calculate the child's dose and the amount to administer for each dose and for a 24-hour period.

The CPS states that a child's dose of:

21. Cephalexin monohydrate (Keflex) is 50 mg/kg administered in equal doses q.6h. Cephalexin monohydrate suspension is available in 5 mL = 250 mg. The child weighs 20 kg.

22. Furosemide (Lasix) is 1 mg/kg administered in equal doses b.i.d. Furosemide oral solution is available in 25-mL bottles with 1 mL = 10 mg. The child weighs 20 kg.

23. Ampicillin sodium (Ampicin) is 50 mg/kg administered in equal doses q.6h. Ampicillin sodium suspension is available in 5 mL = 125 mg. The child weighs 12 kg.

24. Phenytoin (Dilantin) is 5 mg/kg divided equally in 2 or 3 doses, to a maximum of 300 mg. Phenytoin suspension is available in 5 mL = 30 mg. The child weighs 17 kg. Calculate for administration b.i.d.

25. Acetaminophen (Tylenol) is 10 mg/kg (minimum) — divided in equal doses — q.4-6h, not to exceed 65 mg/kg/24 h. Acetaminophen drops are available in 0.8 mL = 80 mg. The child weighs 9 kg. Calculate for administration q.6h.

CHAPTER 5:
PARENTERAL DOSAGES

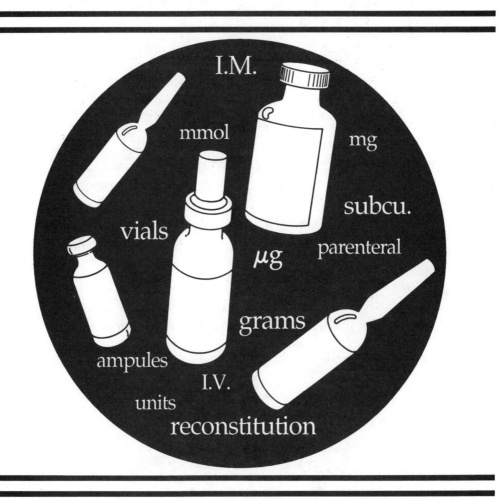

CHAPTER 5

Objectives

1. The student will be able to define and distinguish among the various methods of parenteral administration.

2. The student will demonstrate the ability to calculate accurately the amount of parenteral medication to administer for one dose and for a 24-hour period.

3. The student will be able to apply the medication formulae in reconstitution of single and multiple-dose vials.

4. The student will demonstrate the ability to calculate accurately a child's dose of parenteral medication.

PARENTERAL DOSAGES

The term *parenteral* denotes administration of medication via any route other than the alimentary canal. The parenteral route is used when medications cannot be administered orally or when quick therapeutic action is required.

Parenteral medications are absorbed into the bloodstream faster than oral medications. The amount of medication administered parenterally is usually small, with the exception of intravenous infusions.

Common methods of parenteral administration include:

A. *Intravenous* (I.V.)—into the vein

B. *Intramuscular (I.M.)*—into the muscle

C. *Subcutaneous* (S.C. or subcu.)—into the tissue just below the skin.

Forms of parenteral medications include:

A. Liquids

B. Powders

C. Tablets

Liquids are available in single-dose ampules, single-dose vials, multiple-dose vials, and pre-measured syringes and cartridges. An ampule (ampoule) is a sealed glass container. A vial is a glass container with a rubber stopper (Figure 5-1).

Powders are available in ampules and vials. The powder is dissolved with sterile distilled water to provide an injectable solution.

Tablets can be dissolved in a liquid to provide an injectable solution. These are rarely used today and in most situations would be prepared by a pharmacist.

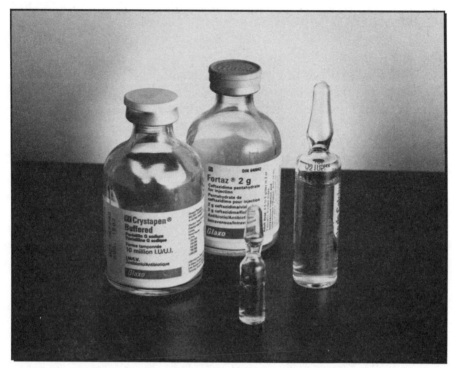

Figure 5-1: Ampules and vials.

Parenteral medications are prepared and administered using syringes. Syringes calibrated in millilitres vary in size, including 3 mL, 5 mL, and 10 mL. The 3-mL syringe is commonly used. Each calibration on this syringe represents 0.1 mL (Figure 5-2).

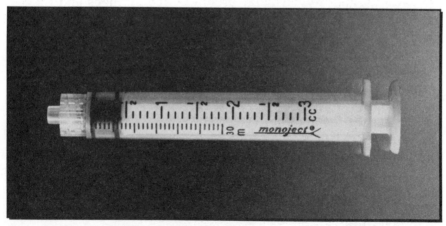

Figure 5-2: Standard 3-mL syringe.

To CALCULATE PARENTERAL DOSES from AMPULES and VIALS:

The formula for calculating the amount of parenteral medication to be administered is the same formula used for oral medications.

$$\frac{\text{DOSE DESIRED}}{\text{DOSE ON HAND}} \times \text{DRUG FORM} = \text{AMOUNT TO ADMINISTER}$$

When calculating parenteral medication, the dose on hand may be stated in:

1. micrograms (μg or mcg)
2. milligrams (mg)
3. grams (g)
4. units (U)
5. millimoles (mmol)

NOTE: Potassium chloride may be ordered in milliequivalents (mEq), which is not a metric unit. The metric equivalent is the millimole (mmol). For example, 20 mEq of KCl is the same as 20 mmol of KCl.

The drug form may be stated in:

A. litres (L)

B. millilitres (mL)

NOTE: As stated in Chapter 4, when using the above formula, remember:

A. The *dose desired* and the *dose on hand* must be expressed in like terms.

B. The *drug form* is always equivalent to the *dose on hand*.

C.   Recheck your calculations if the *amount to administer* is unrealistic.

D.   The words *drug* and *medication* are interchangeable.

> *EXAMPLE #1:* The physician's order reads:
>
> morphine 10 mg I.M. q.4h p.r.n.
>
> Morphine sulfate (Morphine) is available in an ampule labelled 1 mL = 10 mg. How many mL will be administered for each dose?

METHOD #1

$$\frac{\text{Dose Desired}}{\text{Dose on Hand}} \times \text{Drug Form} = \text{Amount to Administer}$$

$$\frac{10 \text{ mg}}{10 \text{ mg}} \times 1 \text{ mL} =$$

$10\overline{)10} = 1$

$1 \times 1 \text{ mL} = 1 \text{ mL}$

METHOD #2

10 mg = 1 mL

10 mg = X mL

10 mg : 1 mL : : 10 mg : X mL

$10 \times X = 1 \times 10$

$10X = 10$

$X = {}^{10}/_{10}$

$X = 1 \text{ mL}$

There will be 1 mL administered for each dose.

EXAMPLE #2: The physician's order reads:

Prostigmin 250 μg S.C. q.4h

Neostigmine (Prostigmin) is available in a 10-mL vial labelled 1 mL = 0.5 mg. How many mL will be administered for each dose?

NOTE: The *dose desired* is in micrograms and the *dose on hand* is in milligrams. The first step in this problem is to change milligrams to micrograms.

1 mg = 1 000 µg
0.5 mg = X µg

Set up a ratio

1 mg : 1 000 µg : : 0.5 mg : X µg

1 x X = 1 000 x 0.5

1X = 500

X = $^{500}/_1$

X = 500 µg

Or

Move the decimal three places to the right.
0.5 mg = 500 µg

METHOD #1

$$\frac{\text{Dose Desired}}{\text{Dose on Hand}} \times \text{Drug Form} = \text{Amount to Administer}$$

$$\frac{250\ \mu g}{500\ \mu g} \times 1\ mL =$$

$$500\ \overline{)\ 250} = 500\ \overline{)\ 250.0}^{.5} = 0.5$$

0.5 x 1 mL = 0.5 mL

METHOD #2

500 μg = 1 mL

250 μg = X mL

500 μg : 1 mL : : 250 μg : X mL

500 x X = 1 x 250

500X = 250

X = $^{250}/_{500}$

X = 0.5 mL

There will be 0.5 mL administered for each dose.

Remember that the dose on hand is an equivalent to the drug form; therefore, 1 mL would be the correct choice for the drug form from the label information.

EXAMPLE #3: The physician's order reads:

Garamycin 60 mg I.M. b.i.d.

Gentamicin sulfate (Garamycin) is available in a 2-mL vial labelled 2 mL = 80 mg. How many mL will be administered for each dose? How many mL will be administered in a 24-hour period?

METHOD #1

$$\frac{\text{Dose Desired}}{\text{Dose on Hand}} \text{ x Drug Form } = \text{ Amount to Administer}$$

$$\frac{60 \text{ mg}}{80 \text{ mg}} \text{ x 2 mL } =$$

AN IMPORTANT POINT TO REMEMBER: The drug form is NOT always 1.

$$80 \overline{)60} = 80 \overline{)60.00}^{.75} = 0.75$$

0.75 x 2 mL = 1.5 mL

There will be 1.5 mL administered for each dose.

b.i.d. = 2 times per day = 2 times in 24 hours

1.5 mL x 2 = 3.0 mL = 3 mL

3 mL will be administered in a 24-hour period.

AN IMPORTANT POINT TO REMEMBER: Fractions are not used in the metric system.

EXAMPLE #4:   The physician's order reads:

Phenergan 50 mg I.V. stat.

Promethazine HCl (Phenergan) is available in an ampule labelled 1 mL = 25 mg. How many mL will be administered for each dose?

METHOD #2

25 mg = 1 mL
50 mg = X mL

25 mg : 1 mL : : 50 mg : X mL

25 x X = 1 x 50

25X = 50

X = $^{50}/_{25}$

X = 2 mL

There will be 2 mL administered for each dose.

NOTE: See Appendix E for answers to questions in this chapter.

Calculate the number of mL administered for each dose and for a 24-hour period:

1. Diphenhydramine HCl (Benadryl) 25 mg I.M. q.6h p.r.n. The medication is available in a 10-mL vial labelled 1 mL = 50 mg.

2. Haloperidol (Haldol) 2.5 mg I.M. stat. The medication is available in a 1-mL ampule containing 5 mg.

3. Dimenhydrinate (Gravol) 25 mg I.M. q.4h p.r.n. The medication is available in a 1-mL single-dose vial containing 50 mg.

4. Cyanocobalamin (vitamin B_{12}) 30 µg subcu. o.d. x 3 days. The medication is available in a 10-mL ampule containing 100 µg (mcg).

5. Furosemide (Lasix) 50 mg I.V. stat. The medication is available in a 2-mL ampule containing 20 mg.

6. Pethidine HCl (Demerol) 50 mg I.M. q.6h p.r.n. The medication is available in a 1-mL ampule containing 100 mg.

7. Hydroxyzine HCl (Atarax) 50 mg I.M. 45 min pre-op. The medication is available in a 1-mL single-dose vial containing 50 mg.

8. Cimetidine (Tagamet) 0.3 g I.V. q.6h. The medication is available in a 2-mL ampule containing 300 mg.

9. Diazepam (Valium) 5 mg I.M. h.s. p.r.n. The medication is available in 2-mL ampule containing 10 mg.

10. Digoxin (Lanoxin) 0.125 mg I.V. o.d. The medication is available in a 2-mL ampule containing 0.25 mg in 1 mL.

To CALCULATE PARENTERAL DOSES from RECONSTITUTED MEDICATIONS:

Many medications are not stable in storage if they are prepared in solution. For this reason, various medications are supplied in powder form in ampules and single- or multiple-dose vials. Antibiotics are commonly found in this form.

Instructions accompany the medications, giving the amount of diluent required to dissolve the powder. To avoid error, it is most important to follow the label directions PRECISELY. This process of dissolving the powder is called *reconstitution.*

To reconstitute antibiotics, sterile distilled water is generally used as a diluent.

EXAMPLE #1: The physician's order reads:

Cephalothin poduim 500 mg I.V. q.6h

Cephalothin sodium (Keflin) is available in a 1-g vial. Instructions state, "add 4.6 mL of sterile water to yield a total volume of 5 mL." How many mL will be administered for each dose?

The first step is to convert grams to milligrams. Move the decimal place three places to the right.

1 g = 1 000 mg

METHOD #1

$$\frac{\text{Dose Desired}}{\text{Dose on Hand}} \times \text{Drug Form} = \text{Amount to Administer}$$

$$\frac{500 \text{ mg}}{1\,000 \text{ mg}} \times 5 \text{ mL} =$$

$$1\,000\overline{)500} = 1\,000\overline{)500.0}^{.5} = 0.5$$

0.5 x 5 mL = 2.5 mL

METHOD #2

$1\,000$ mg $=$ 5 mL

500 mg $=$ X mL

$1\,000$ mg : 5 mL : : 500 mg : X mL

$1\,000$ x X $=$ 5 x 500

$1\,000$ X $=$ $2\,500$

X $=$ $^{2\,500}/_{1\,000}$

X $=$ 2.5

There will be 2.5 mL administered for each dose.

EXAMPLE #2: The physician's order reads:

Ampicin 500 mg I.M. q.6h

Ampicillin (Ampicin) is available in a 1-g vial. Instructions state, "add 3.5 mL of sterile water to yield a total volume of 4 mL." How many mL will be administered for each dose? How many mL will be administered in a 24-hour period?
The first step is to convert grams to milligrams.

1 g $=$ $1\,000$ mg

METHOD #1

$$\frac{\text{Dose Desired}}{\text{Dose on Hand}} \times \text{Drug Form} = \text{Amount to Administer}$$

$$\frac{500 \text{ mg}}{1\,000 \text{ mg}} \times 4 \text{ mL} =$$

NOTE: An alternative to long division is first to cancel zeroes, reduce to lowest terms and convert to a decimal fraction.

$$\frac{500}{1\,000} = \frac{1}{2}$$

$$2\overline{)\,1} = 2\overline{)\,1.0}^{\;.5} = 0.5$$

0.5 x 4 mL = 2.0 mL = 2 mL

METHOD #2

1 000 mg = 4 mL
500 mg = X mL

1 000 mg : 4 mL : : 500 mg : X mL

1 000 x X = 4 x 500

1 000 X = 2 000

$X = {}^{2\,000}/_{1\,000}$

X = 2 mL

There will be 2 mL administered for each dose.

q.6h = every 6 hours = 4 times in 24 hours

2 mL x 4 = 8 mL

8 mL will be administered in a 24-hour period

EXAMPLE #3: The physician's order reads:

Penicillin G sodium 300 000 U I.V. q.8h

Penicillin G sodium (Crystapen) is available in a 1 000 000-U vial. Instructions state, "add 10 mL of sterile water." How many mL will be administered for each dose?

METHOD #1

$$\frac{\text{Dose Desired}}{\text{Dose on Hand}} \times \text{Drug Form} = \text{Amount to Administer}$$

In this example, no total volume is given. Some powders add no volume. In such cases, the *drug form* is the amount of diluent added.

When reconstituting a multiple-strength solution, the most appropriate strength must be chosen.

$$\frac{300\,000\ \text{U}}{1\,000\,000\ \text{U}} \times 10\ \text{mL} =$$

$$\frac{300\,000\ \text{U}}{1\,000\,000\ \text{U}} = \frac{3}{10}$$

$$10\overline{)\underset{3.0}{\,.3\,}} = 0.3$$

$$0.3 \times 10\ \text{mL} = 3.0\ \text{mL} = 3\ \text{mL}$$

METHOD #2

1 000 000 U = 10 mL
300 000 U = X mL

1 000 000 U : 10 mL : : 300 000 U : X mL

1 000 000 × X = 10 × 300 000

1 000 000 X = 3 000 000

$$X = \frac{3\,000\,000}{1\,000\,000}$$

$$X = \frac{3}{1}$$

X = 3 mL

There will be 3 mL administered for each dose.

Some medication labels give a smaller ratio to simplify calculations. For example, the above ratio of 1 000 00 units = 10 mL might be given as 100 000 units = 1 mL. Fitting this ratio into the above problem would give the same answer.

METHOD #1

$$\frac{300\,000\ U}{100\,000\ U} \times 1\ mL =$$

$$\frac{300\,000\ U}{100\,000\ U} = \frac{3}{1} = 3$$

$$3 \times 1\ mL = 3\ mL$$

METHOD #2

$$100\,000\ U = 1\ mL$$
$$300\,000\ U = X\ mL$$

$$100\,000\ U : 1\ mL : : 300\,000\ U : X\ mL$$

$$100\,000 \times X = 1 \times 300\,000$$

$$100\,000X = 300\,000$$

$$X = \frac{300\,000}{100\,000} = \frac{3}{1} = 3$$

$$X = 3\ mL$$

There will be 3 mL administered for each dose.

As well as giving a smaller ratio to simplify calculations, certain medication labels may have a dilution table, which gives equivalencies for various concentrations of the medication. The most appropriate one to provide the dose desired is chosen (Figure 5-3). It is important always to read labels carefully for accurate reconstitution.

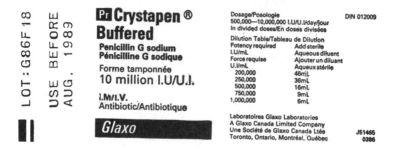

Figure 5-3: Medication label with a dilution table.

AN IMPORTANT POINT TO REMEMBER:

The *dose on hand* and the *drug form* should be equivalent. If the numbers used in these two sections of the formula are not equivalent, the *amount to administer* will be calculated incorrectly.

Calculate the number of mL administered for each dose and for a 24-hour period:

11. Cloxacillin sodium monohydrate (Orbenin) 250 mg I.V. q.6h. The medication is available in a 250-mg vial. Instructions are to add 1.9 mL of sterile water to yield 2 mL.

12. Cefazolin sodium (Ancef) 0.5 g I.V. q.8h x 2 doses. The medication is available in a 500-mg vial. Instructions are to add 2 mL of sterile water to yield 2.2 mL.

13. Tetracycline HCl (Tetracyn) 500 mg I.V. stat. The medication is available in a 250-mg vial. Instructions are to add 1.8 mL of sterile water to yield 2 mL.

14. Ampicillin (Ampicin) 250 mg I.V. q.6h. The medication is available in a 250-mg vial. Instructions are to add 2 mL of sterile water.

15. Penicillin G sodium (Crystapen) 750 000 U I.V. q.4h. The medication is available in a 5 000 000-U vial. The dilution table on the label reads:

Potency required U per mL	Add sterile aqueous diluent
200 000	23 mL
250 000	18 mL
500 000	8 mL
750 000	4.6 mL
1 000 000	3 mL

To CALCULATE PARENTERAL DOSES for CHILDREN:

The general formula for calculating a child's dose can be used for parenteral medication.

DRUG DOSE x CHILD'S WEIGHT = CHILD'S DOSE
(in mg/kg)   (in kilograms)

EXAMPLE: The CPS states a child's dose of furosemide (Lasix) is 0.5 mg/kg administered in equally divided doses q.12h. Furosemide is available in a multiple-dose 30-mL vial labelled 1 mL = 0.5 mg. Calculate the dose for a child weighing 12 kg. How many mL will be administered for each dose?

0.5 mg/kg x 12 kg = 6.0 mg

Child's dose for a 24-hour period = 6 mg

6 mg in equal doses q.12h =

6 mg ÷ 2 = 3 mg

3 mg will be administered q.12h.

Using the general formula to calculate the amount to administer:

METHOD #1

$$\frac{\text{Dose Desired}}{\text{Dose on Hand}} \times \text{Drug Form} = \text{Amount to Administer}$$

$$\frac{3 \text{ mg}}{0.5 \text{ mg}} \times 1 \text{ mL} =$$

$$0.5 \overline{)3} = 5 \overline{)30.0}^{6.0} = 6$$

$$6 \times 1 \text{ mL} = 6 \text{ mL}$$

METHOD #2

0.5 mg = 1 mL
3 mg = X mL

0.5 mg : 1 mL : : 3 mg : X mL

0.5 mg x X mL = 1 mL x 3 mg

0.5X = 3

X = $^3/_{0.5}$

X = 6 mL

There will be 6 mL administered for each dose.

Calculate the child's dose and the number of mL to administer for each dose and for a 24-hour period where applicable:

The CPS states a child's dose of:

16. Diazepam (Valium) is 1 mg/4.5 kg. The medication is available in 2-mL ampules containing 5 mg per mL. The child weighs 18 kg.

17. Gentamicin sulfate (Garamycin) is 6 mg/kg in equal doses q.8h. The medication is available in 2-mL vials containing 40 mg per mL. The child weighs 6 kg.

18. Pancuronium bromide (Pavulon) is 60 µg/kg. The medication is available in 2-mL ampules containing 2 mg per mL. The child weighs 16 kg.

19. Digoxin (Lanoxin) is 0.025 mg/kg. The medication is available in 2-mL ampules containing 0.25 mg. The child weighs 12 kg.

20. Pethidine HCl (Demerol) is 1.1 mg/kg q.4h. The medication is available in a 1-mL ampule containing 50 mg. The child weighs 10 kg.

CHAPTER 6:
INSULIN HEPARIN
AND I.V. ADDITIVES

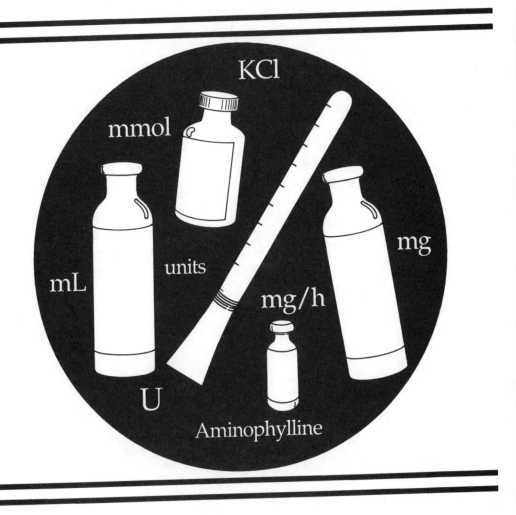

CHAPTER 6

Objectives

1. The student will demonstrate the ability to calculate accurately the amount of insulin and heparin to administer for one dose.

2. The student will demonstrate the ability to calculate I.V. additives accurately.

3. The student will demonstrate the ability to calculate accurately intravenous infusions of heparin and aminophylline.

INSULIN DOSAGES

The major therapeutic use for *insulin* is the treatment of *diabetes*. A number of insulin preparations are available today (Appendix N). Insulins are available in 10-mL multiple-dose vials. The strength of insulins has been standardized to 100 U per mL. Most insulin preparations are administered subcutaneously. Any regular unmodified insulin can also be administered intravenously.

Insulin is generally prepared in an insulin syringe, which is calibrated in units. A 1-mL insulin syringe is calibrated in 100 units. A 0.5-mL insulin syringe is calibrated in 50 units (Figure 6-1). Combinations of insulins are frequently mixed in one syringe. When combining short- and long-acting insulins, the short-acting insulin is prepared first.

Insulin is ordered in units. Formulae are not required to calculate the amount of insulin to administer when an insulin syringe is used. The dose desired and the syringe are in units; therefore, the *amount to administer* is actually the *dose desired.*

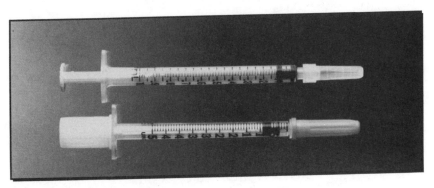

Figure 6-1: Insulin syringes.

To CALCULATE INSULIN DOSES when a standard syringe calibrated in mL is used:

The formula for calculating the amount of insulin to be administered is the same formula used for oral medications.

$$\frac{\text{DOSE DESIRED}}{\text{DOSE ON HAND}} \times \text{DRUG FORM} = \text{AMOUNT TO ADMINISTER}$$

When calculating insulin, the *dose desired* and the *dose on hand* will be stated in units (U). The *drug form* will be stated in millilitres (mL).

EXAMPLE #1: The physician's order reads:

Lente insulin 16U
CZI 36 u   } subcu. a.c. q.a.m.

Each insulin is available in a 10-mL vial labelled 1 mL = 100 U. How many mL will be administered for each dose?

Lente insulin

METHOD #1

$$\frac{\text{Dose Desired}}{\text{Dose on Hand}} \times \text{Drug Form} = \text{Amount to Administer}$$

$$\frac{16\,\text{U}}{100\,\text{U}} \times 1\,\text{mL} =$$

$$100\,\overline{)16} = 100\overline{)\,16.00}^{\,.16} = 0.16$$

$$0.16 \times 1\ \text{mL} = 0.16\ \text{mL}$$

METHOD #2

100 U = 1 mL
16 U = X mL

100 U : 1 mL : : 16 U : X mL

100 x X = 1 x 16

100X = 16

X = 16/100

X = 0.16 mL

NOTE: Insulin calculations are not rounded to one decimal place because administration of the incorrect dose may result in adverse effects.

CZI insulin

METHOD #1

$$\frac{\text{Dose Desired}}{\text{Dose on Hand}} \times \text{Drug Form} = \text{Amount to Administer}$$

$$\frac{36\,U}{100\,U} \times 1\,mL =$$

$$100 \,\overline{)\,36} = 100 \,\overline{)\,36.00}^{\,.36} = 0.36$$

$$0.36 \times 1\ mL = 0.36\ mL$$

NOTE: Some insulins and syringes may be supplied in cc. Remember that 1 cc = 1 mL.

METHOD #2

100 U = 1 mL
36 U = X mL

100 U : 1 mL : : 36 U : X mL

100 x X = 1 x 36

$X = {}^{36}/_{100}$

X = 0.36 mL

Each day 0.16 mL of lente insulin and 0.36 mL of CZI insulin will be administered for a total injection of 0.52 mL.

NOTE: See Appendix F for answers to questions in this chapter.

Calculate the number of mL to be administered for each dose:

1. Initard insulin 40 U subcu. $^1/_2$ h a.c. q.a.m. The insulin is available in a 10-mL multiple-dose vial labelled 1 mL = 100 U.

2. Mixtard 35 U S.C. @ 07:30 o.d. & Mixtard 10 U S.C. @ 16:30 o.d. The insulin is available in a 10-mL multiple-dose vial labelled 1 mL = 100 U.

3. Velosulin Human insulin 12 U subcu. stat. The insulin is available in a 10-mL multiple-dose vial labelled 1 mL = 100 U.

4. Humulin-R insulin 10 U subcu. 45 min a.c. q.a.m. The insulin is available in a 10-mL multiple-dose vial labelled 1 mL = 100 U.

5. NPH insulin 35 U and Novolin-Toronto insulin 25 U S.C. 30 min a.c. q.a.m. Each insulin is available in a 10-mL multiple-dose vial labelled 1 mL = 100 U.

SUBCUTANEOUS AND I.V. HEPARIN

Heparin is also ordered in units. It is often prepared in an insulin syringe, because doses of less than 1 mL are usually ordered. Heparin is available in concentrations of 1 000 U/mL and 10 000 U/mL, as well as a flush solution of 100 U/mL for heparin-locks. When an insulin syringe is used for the larger concentrations, the number of mL to administer is calculated, and the syringe markings in mL (cc) are used in place of U.

To CALCULATE HEPARIN DOSES:

EXAMPLE :   The physician's order reads:

Heparin 5 000 U S.C. q. 12h

Heparin sodium (Heparin) is available in a 10-mL vial labelled 1 mL = 10 000 U. How many mL will be administered for each dose?

METHOD #1

$$\frac{\text{Dose Desired}}{\text{Dose on Hand}} \times \text{Drug Form} = \text{Amount to Administer}$$

$$\frac{5\,000\ U}{10\,000\ U} \times 1\ mL =$$

$$10\overline{)\ 5} = 10\overline{)\ 5.0}^{\,0.5} = 0.5$$

$$0.5 \times 1\ mL = 0.5\ mL$$

METHOD #2

10 000 U = 1 mL
5 000 U = X mL

10 000 U : 1 mL : : 5 000 U : X mL

10 000 x X = 1 x 5 000

10 000 X = 5 000

$X = {}^{5\,000}/_{10\,000}$

X = 0.5 mL

There will be 0.5 mL of heparin administered for each dose.

Calculate the number of mL to be administered for each dose:

6. Heparin 6 000 U I.V. push. The medication is available in a 10-mL multiple-dose vial labelled 1 mL = 10 000 U.

7. Heparin 3 000 U subcu. q.12h. The medication is available in a 10-mL multiple-dose vial labelled 1 mL = 10 000 U.

8. Flush Heparin-lock with 100 U Hepalean-Lok solution b.i.d. The medication is available in a 10-mL multiple-dose vial labelled 1 mL = 100 U.

9. Heparin 5 000 U subcu. 2 h pre-op. The medication is available in a 10-mL multiple-dose vial labelled 1 mL = 10 000 U.

10. Heparin 7 000 U I.V. push. The medication is available in a 10-mL multiple-dose vial labelled 1 mL = 1 000 U.

I.V. ADDITIVES

Certain medications are often administered in large volumes of intravenous solution. Common I.V. additives include potassium chloride (KCl), aminophylline, heparin, and insulin. Many additive orders are written in ratios of medication to I.V. solution (for example, "Add 20 mmol KCl to each litre of I.V. solution."). Other orders are written in ratios of medication to time. For example, "aminophylline 35 mg/h in 500 mL I.V. D5W."

To CALCULATE amounts of I.V. ADDITIVES:

The formula for oral medications is again used.

$$\frac{\text{Dose Desired}}{\text{Dose on Hand}} \times \text{Drug Form} = \text{Amount to Administer}$$

EXAMPLE #1: The physician's order reads:

add 10 u Toronto insulin to 1 000 mL I.V. N/s

Novolin-Toronto insulin is available in a 10-mL multiple-dose vial containing 100 U per mL.

METHOD #1

$$\frac{\text{Dose Desired}}{\text{Dose on Hand}} \times \text{Drug Form} = \text{Amount to Administer}$$

$$\frac{10\ U}{100\ U} \times 1\ mL =$$

$$100\ \overline{)\ 10} = 100\ \overline{)\ 10.0}^{\ .1} = 0.1$$

$$0.1 \times 1\ mL = 0.1\ mL$$

METHOD #2

100 U = 1 mL
10 U = X mL

100 U : 1 mL : : 10 U : X mL

100 x X = 1 x 10

100X = 10

X = $^{10}/_{100}$

X = 0.1 mL

There will be 0.1 mL of Novolin-Toronto insulin added to 1 000 mL of I.V. normal saline.

EXAMPLE #2: The physician's order reads:

Add 30 mmol KCl/L of I.V. solution

Prepare I.V. Ringer's lactate solution 500 mL. Potassium chloride (KCl) is available in a 20-mL single-dose vial containing 40 mmol.

The order is written for preparation of a litre of I.V. solution. The I.V. to be prepared is 500 mL. The first step is to calculate how many mmol are required for 500 mL.

Remember to convert 1 L to 1 000 mL, then set up a ratio:

1 000 mL = 30 mmol
500 mL = X mmol

1 000 mL : 30 mmol : : 500 mL : X mmol

1 000 x X = 30 x 500

1 000X = 15 000

X = $^{15\,000}/_{1\,000}$

X = 15 mmol

15 mmol of KCl are required for 500 mL

METHOD #1

$$\frac{\text{Dose Desired}}{\text{Dose on Hand}} \times \text{Drug Form} = \text{Amount to Administer}$$

$$\frac{15 \text{ mmol}}{40 \text{ mmol}} \times 20 \text{ mL} =$$

$$40\overline{)\ 15} = 40\ \overset{.375}{\overline{)15.000}} = 0.375$$

$$0.375 \times 20 \text{ mL} = 7.5 \text{ mL}$$

METHOD #2

40 mmol = 20 mL
15 mmol = X mL

40 mmol : 20 mL : : 15 mmol : X mL

40 x X = 20 x 15

40X = 300

X = $300/40$

X = 7.5 mL
There will be 7.5 mL of potassium chloride (KCl) added to 500 mL of I.V. Ringer's lactate solution.

NOTE: Remember that when KCl is ordered in mEq and supplied in mmol, the mEq = mmol. For example, 30 mEq = 30 mmol.

Calculate the amount of I.V. additive required:

11. Potassium chloride 15 mmol/L. Prepare 500 mL of I.V. N/S. Potassium chloride is available in a 10-mL single-dose vial labelled 20 mmol.

12. Iletin Regular 15 U in 1 000 mL of I.V. D5W. Iletin Regular is available in a 10-mL multiple-dose vial labelled 1 mL = 100 U.

13. KCl 20 mEq/L. Prepare 1 L of I.V. 0.9% sodium chloride. KCl is available in a 20-mL single-dose vial labelled 40 mmol.

14. Novalin-Toronto insulin 25 U in 1 000 mL of I.V. 10% dextrose and water. Novolin-Toronto insulin is available in a 10-mL multiple-dose vial labelled 1 mL = 100 U.

15. Potassium chloride 10 mmol/500 mL. Prepare 500 mL of I.V. 2/3 & 1/3. Potassium chloride is available in a 10-mL single-dose vial labelled 20 mmol.

To CALCULATE I.V. HEPARIN and AMINOPHYLLINE:

Intravenous heparin may be calculated and prepared using different methods. The dose is generally ordered in units per hour. The first method calculates the number of millilitres required to provide the hourly dose. Once calculated, the amount of heparin may be added hourly to the intravenous infusion set.

Another method prepares an intravenous solution for continuous infusion. These infusions are often referred to as drips, for example, "a heparin drip." To use this method, the *hourly dose, hourly volume,* and *total volume* of the intravenous solution must be calculated.

Proportions can also be used to calculate the hourly dose in millilitres and the total dosage and amount of heparin to be added to the intravenous solution for a continuous infusion.

NOTE: Various ratios may be used to calculate the number of mL required. Always ensure that the ratio is a given equivalency.

Aminophylline is generally ordered in mg/h at a specified rate. It may be administered as an hourly dose, but is generally prepared as a continuous infusion.

Intravenous infusions may be controlled by an electronic infusion device, such as a controller or pump. Caution should be taken when using these devices, especially when they are temporarily stopped. The open clamp should be partially closed and the flow rate manually regulated before leaving the infusion.

EXAMPLE #1 The physician's order reads:

Heparin 750 U I.V. q.1h. Infuse I.V. N/S @ 50 mL/h.

Heparin is available in a 10-mL vial labelled 1 mL = 1 000 units. How many mL of Heparin will be added for each dose? How many mL of Heparin will be added to 500 mL of I.V. N/S to prepare a continuous infusion?

To calculate an hourly dose:

METHOD #1

$$\frac{\text{Dose Desired}}{\text{Dose on Hand}} \times \text{Drug Form} = \text{Amount to Administer}$$

$$\frac{750\ U}{1\ 000\ U} \times 1\ mL =$$

$$100\ \overline{)75} = 100\ \overline{)\ 75.00}^{\ .75} = 0.75$$

$$0.75 \times 1\ mL = 0.75\ mL$$

METHOD #2

$1\ 000\ U = 1\ mL$

$750\ U = X\ mL$

$1\ 000\ U : 1\ mL :: 750\ U : X\ mL$

$1\ 000 \times X = 1 \times 750$

$1\ 000X = 750$

$X = {}^{750}/_{1\ 000}$

$X = 0.75\ mL$

There will be 0.75 mL of Heparin (1 000 U = 1 mL) added for each dose of 750 U of Heparin. This is the amount of Heparin that may be added hourly to the intravenous infusion set.

To prepare a continuous infusion:

METHOD #1 :

A. Calculate the hourly dose using one of the preceding methods.
B. Note the hourly volume, which is the I.V. rate per hour.
C. Note the total volume of I.V. solution required.
D. Divide the total volume by the hourly volume to obtain the number of doses in the total volume.
E. Multiply the hourly dose by the number of doses in the total volume to obtain the number of mL of Heparin to be added to the total volume.

To prepare the infusion ordered in Example #1:

A. The hourly dose = 0.75 mL

B. The hourly volume = 50 mL/h

C. The total volume = 500 mL

D. $\dfrac{500 \text{ mL}}{50 \text{ mL/h}} = 5\overline{\smash{\big)}50}^{\displaystyle 10} = 10 \text{ h}$

If the hourly rate is maintained at 50 mL/h, 500 mL of I.V. N/S will infuse in 10 hours. To prepare a continuous infusion, 10 doses of Heparin will be added to the 500 mL.

E. 0.75 mL x 10 doses = 7.5 mL
There will be 7.5 mL of Heparin (1 000 U = 1 mL) added to 500 mL of I.V. N/S to prepare a continuous infusion of 750 U/h.

METHOD #2

A. Set up a proportion to calculate the dosage of Heparin required for the total volume of I.V. solution. The physician ordered 750 U/h at a rate of 50 mL/h.

50 mL = 750 U

500 mL = X U

50 mL : 750 U : : 500 mL : X U

50 x X = 750 x 500

50X = 375 000

$X = {}^{375\,000}/_{50}$

X = 7 500 U

There will be 7 500 U of Heparin added to 500 mL of I.V. N/S.

B. Set up a second proportion, using the dosage required for the total volume of I.V. solution, to calculate the number of mL of Heparin required to prepare a continuous infusion. The vial contains 1 000 U/mL.

1 000 U/mL

1 000 U = 1 mL
7 500 U = X mL

1 000 U : 1 mL : : 7 500 U : X mL

1 000 x X = 1 x 7 500

1 000X = 7 500

$X = {}^{7\,500}/_{1\,000}$

X = 7.5 mL

There will be 7.5 mL of Heparin (1 000 U = 1 mL) added to 500 mL of I.V. N/S to prepare a continuous infusion of 750 U/h.

EXAMPLE #2: The physician's order reads:

Aminophylline 35 mg/h @ 35 mL/h in I.V. D5W 500mL

Aminophylline is available in a 10-mL
ampule labelled 1 mL = 50 mg. How many
mL of aminophylline will be added for each
dose?

To calculate an hourly dose:

METHOD #1

$$\frac{\text{Dose Desired}}{\text{Dose on Hand}} \times \text{Drug Form} = \text{Amount to Administer}$$

$$\frac{35 \text{ mg}}{50 \text{ mg}} \times 1 \text{ mL} =$$

$$50 \overline{)\, 35} = 50 \overline{)\, 35.0}^{.7} = 0.7$$

0.7 X 1 mL = 0.7 mL

METHOD #2

50 mg = 1 mL
35 mg = X mL

50 mg : 1 mL : : 35 mg : X mL

50 x X = 1 x 35

50X = 35

X = $^{35}/_{50}$

X = 0.7 mL
There will be 0.7 mL of aminophylline
(50 mg = 1 mL) added for each dose of
35 mg of aminophylline. This is the amount
of aminophylline that may be added hourly
to the intravenous infusion set.

To prepare a continuous infusion of aminophylline, 500 mg of aminophylline (500 mg = 10 mL) is commonly added to 500 mL of I.V. solution. This infusion provides 1 mg of aminophylline per mL of I.V. solution. Physicians using this method increase or decrease the hourly dose of aminophylline by ordering changes in the rate per hour of the infusion. The dosage in 500 mL remains 1 mL = 1 mg.

To prepare Example #2 according to this method, aminophylline 500 mg would be added to I.V. D5W 500 mL. The rate per hour of the infusion would be 35 mL. If the physician increased the hourly dose to 40 mg/h, the rate per hour of the infusion would be increased to 40 mL, and the I.V. solution would remain unchanged.

This method provides a standard, as well as a workable, ratio. If this standard is not used, the methods for preparing heparin infusions can be applied.

NOTE: The methods for preparing continuous heparin infusions are accurate when the ordered rate per hour is 50 mL or a rate that divides evenly into the total volume. Other rates will not provide accurate calculations because answers will have to be rounded off. In such cases, the ordering physician should be consulted before the infusion is prepared.

Calculate the number of mL to be added hourly to each I.V. and where appropriate prepare a continuous infusion:

16. Add 700 U of Heparin to 50 mL of I.V. N/S q.1h. Prepare I.V. N/S 500 mL. The medication is available in a 10-mL multiple-dose vial labelled 1 mL = 1 000 U.

17. Heparin 600 U/h I.V. Infuse 500 mL of I.V. N/S at 50 mL/h. The medication is available in a 10-mL multiple-dose vial labelled 1 mL = 1 000 U.

18. Heparin 450 U I.V. q.1h in I.V. N/S 500 mL @ 50 mL/h. The medication is available in a 10-mL multiple-dose vial labelled 1 mL = 1 000 U.

19. Aminophylline 40 mg/h in I.V. normal saline @ 40 mL/h. The medication is available in a 10-mL ampule containing 500 mg.

20. Aminophylline 30 mg/h in I.V. D5W at 30 mL/h. The medication is available in a 10-mL ampule with 1 mL = 50 mg.

CHAPTER 7:
INTRAVENOUS FLOW RATES

drops/millilitre

DIOW   mL/min

I.V. R/L @1.5 mL/min

electronic infusion devices   5%D/W

I.V. 2/3 &1/3 @ 100 mL/h

1 mL=10gtts.

infusion sets   24:00   XXI

gtts./mL   Heparin

5% dextrose +1/2 normal saline

Ringer's lactate

20 gtts./mL   5% D/S

microdrops

normal saline

CHAPTER 7

Objectives

1. The student will demonstrate an understanding of the term *flow rate*, its influencing factors, and the term *drop factor*.

2. The student will demonstrate the ability to calculate I.V. flow rates accurately.

3. The student will demonstrate the ability to calculate hourly I.V. rates accurately.

INTRAVENOUS FLOW RATES

The *flow rate* is the number of drops per minute (gtts./min) a fluid is administered intravenously. The *drop factor* is the number of drops per millilitre (gtts./mL) of fluid administered.

Different I.V. infusion sets have different drop factors, which are found on the infusion set package. The most common drop factors are 10, 15, 20, and 60 drops per millilitre.

When administering I.V. solutions to children, a buretrol infusion set is generally used. The drop factor for a buretrol is 60 gtts./mL. These drops are referred to as microdrops and allow more accurate control of the smaller volumes generally ordered for children.

To ensure accurate infusion, it is recommended that infusion rates be checked every 15 minutes.

Factors that affect the rate of an infusion include the

- body size,
- age,
- patency of the needle,
- need for fluids,
- type of fluid administered,
- position of the needle,
- movement of the body part where the needle is inserted,
- condition of the cardiac or renal system,
- position of the bed or the I.V. pole,
- position of the regulating clamp, and
- set rate of an electronic infusion device.

To CALCULATE the FLOW RATE:

A general formula is used to calculate the flow rate (Figure 7-1).

$$\frac{\text{DROP FACTOR (gtts./mL)} \times \text{RATE PER HOUR (mL/h)}}{60 \text{ MINUTES/HOUR}} = \text{FLOW RATE (gtts./min)}$$

Figure 7-1: General formula for calculating flow rates.

EXAMPLE #1: The physician's order reads:

I.V. ²/3 + ⅓ @ 120 mL/h

The drop factor for the I.V. infusion set is 60 drops per millilitre. What is the flow rate?

$$\frac{\text{DROP FACTOR} \times \text{RATE PER HOUR}}{60 \text{ MINUTES/HOUR}} = \text{FLOW RATE (gtts./min)}$$

(gtts./mL) (mL/h)

$$\frac{60 \text{ gtts./mL} \times 120 \text{ mL/h}}{60 \text{ min/h}} =$$

$$\frac{7\,200}{60} =$$

$$6\,\overline{)\,720} = 120$$

Flow rate = 120 gtts./min

EXAMPLE #2: The physician's order reads:

I.V. D5W @ 200 mL/h

The drop factor for the I.V. infusion set is 10 gtts./mL. What is the flow rate?

$$\frac{\text{DROP FACTOR} \times \text{RATE PER HOUR}}{60 \text{ MINUTES/HOUR}} = \text{FLOW RATE (gtts./min)}$$

(gtts./mL) (mL/h)

$$\frac{10 \text{ gtts./mL} \times 200 \text{ mL/h}}{60 \text{ min/h}} =$$

$$\frac{2\,000}{60} =$$

$$6\,\overline{)\,200} = 6\,\overline{)\,200.0} = 33.3 = 33$$

Flow rate = 33 gtts./min

NOTE: Decimal answers are not acceptable for flow rates because a portion of a drop cannot be obtained.

NOTE: See Appendix G for answers to questions in this chapter.

Calculate the flow rates:

1. I.V. Ringer's lactate solution @ 140 mL/h. The drop factor of the I.V. infusion set is 20 gtts./mL.

2. I.V. 5% dextrose and 0.45% normal saline at 100 mL/h. The I.V. infusion set delivers 60 drops/mL.

3. I.V. 10% dextrose and water at 150 mL/h. The I.V. infusion set delivers 10 gtts./mL.

4. I.V. 2/3 & 1/3 @ 200 mL/h for the next 3 h then decrease the rate to 125 mL/h. The drop factor of the I.V. infusion set is 20 gtts./mL.

5. I.V. normal saline 75 mL over the next hour, then increase to 125 mL/h. The drop factor of the I.V. infusion set is 60 gtts./mL.

The $\dfrac{mL/h}{60\ min/h}$ as used in the previous formula may be replaced by the metric standard of millilitres per minute (mL/min) to give a metric standard formula (Figure 7-2).

DROP FACTOR x MILLILITRES PER MINUTE = FLOW RATE
  (gtts./mL)   (mL/min)   (gtts./min)

Figure 7-2: Metric standard formula for flow rates.

The following examples use the metric standard formula.

EXAMPLE #1: The physician's order reads:

I.V. ²/₃+⅓ @ 2 mL/min

The drop factor for the I.V. infusion set is 60 drops per millilitre. What is the flow rate?

DROP FACTOR x	MILLILITRES PER MINUTE =	FLOW RATE
(gtts./mL)	(mL/min)	(gtts./min)

60 gtts./mL x 2 mL/min =
Flow rate = 120 gtts./min

EXAMPLE #2: The physician's order reads:

I.V. D5W @ 3.3 millilitres per minute

The drop factor for the I.V. infusion set is 10 gtts./mL. What is the flow rate?

DROP FACTOR x	MILLILITRES PER MINUTE	= FLOW RATE
(gtts./mL)	(mL/min)	(gtts./min)

10 gtts./mL x 3.3 mL/min =

33.3 = 33 gtts./min

Flow rate = 33 gtts./min

Calculate the flow rates:

6. I.V. N/S @ 4 mL/min. The drop factor for the I.V. infusion set is 10 drops per millilitre.

7. I.V. D10W @ 3 mL/min. The drop factor for the I.V. infusion set is 60 gtts./mL.

8. I.V. 5% dextrose & 1/2 N/S @ 1.3 mL/min. The I.V. infusion set delivers 20 gtts./mL.

9. I.V. R/L @ 2 mL/min. The I.V. infusion set delivers 10 gtts./mL.

10. I.V. 5% D&S @ 2.5 mL/min. The drop factor for the I.V. infusion set is 60 gtts./mL.

Intravenous solutions may be ordered for a time period other than one hour. For example, "Infuse 500 mL of I.V. ²/₃ & ¹/₃ over 4 h".

To CALCULATE the FLOW RATE when the rate per hour is not ordered, using the GENERAL FORMULA:

A. Calculate the rate per hour by dividing the total volume by the total number of hours.

B. Calculate the flow rate using the general formula.

EXAMPLE: The physician's order reads:

Infuse 540 mL of 10% dextrose + water over 3 hours

The drop factor of the I.V. infusion set is 10 drops per mL.

A. $\dfrac{540 \text{ mL}}{3 \text{ h}}$ = 180 mL/h

Rate per hour = 180 mL/h

B. General formula:

$$\frac{\text{DROP FACTOR (gtts./mL)} \times \text{RATE PER HOUR (mL/h)}}{60 \text{ MINUTES/HOUR}} = \text{FLOW RATE (gtts./min)}$$

$$\frac{10 \text{ gtts./mL} \times 180 \text{ mL/h}}{60 \text{ min/h}} =$$

$$\frac{1\,800}{60} =$$

$6\overline{)180} = 30$

Flow rate = 30 gtts./min

Calculate the flow rates using the general formula:

11. 100 mL of 25% human albumin over 2 hours. The drop factor for the I.V. infusion set is 15 gtts./mL.

12. 75 mL of I.V. D5W over 1/2 hour. The I.V. infusion set delivers 10 gtts./mL.

13. I.V. $^2/_3$ & $^1/_3$, 1 200 mL over 24 hours. The drop factor for the I.V. infusion set is 60 gtts./mL.

14. 1 500 mL of whole blood intravenously over the next 12 hours, followed by 1 000 mL of I.V. N/S over 8 hours. The drop factor for the blood infusion set is 15 gtts./mL. The drop factor for the N/S infusion set is 10 gtts./mL.

15. 750 mL of Ringer's lactate solution over a 10-hour period, followed by 2 000 mL of D5W over a 20-hour period. The drop factor for the I.V. infusion set is 60 gtts./mL.

To CALCULATE the FLOW RATE when the millilitres per minute are not ordered, using the METRIC STANDARD FORMULA:
A. Calculate the millilitres per minute by multiplying the total number of hours by 60 min/h.
B. Divide the total volume by the number obtained in the previous step.
C. Calculate the flow rate using the metric standard formula.
     EXAMPLE: The physician's order reads:
     Infuse 540 mL of 10% dextrose & water over 3 hours
                     The drop factor of the I.V. infusion set is 10 drops per mL.

     A. 3 h x 60 min/h = 180 min

     B. $\dfrac{540 \text{ mL}}{180 \text{ min}}$ = 3 mL/min

C.   Metric standard formula:

DROP FACTOR x MILLILITRES PER MINUTE
$$\frac{\text{(gtts./mL)} \qquad \text{(mL/min)}}{60 \text{ MINUTES/HOUR}} = \text{FLOW RATE (gtts./min)}$$

10 gtts./mL x 3 mL/min =

Flow rate = 30 gtts./min

Calculate the flow rates using the metric standard formula:

16. 3 600 mL of 2/3 & 1/3 intravenously in a 24-hour period. The I.V. infusion set delivers 10 gtts./mL.

17. Ringer's lactate solution 3 000 mL intravenously in 24 hours. The drop factor for the I.V. infusion set is 60 gtts./mL.

18. I.V. 5% dextrose & saline 1 000 mL over the next 5 hours, then 1 000 mL over 10 hours. The drop factor for the I.V. infusion set is 20 gtts./mL.

19. 50 mL of 0.9% sodium chloride I.V. over 20 minutes, then 3 000 mL over 24 hours. The I.V. infusion set delivers 10 gtts./mL.

20. 100 mL of I.V. D5W over 1/2 hour. The drop factor for the I.V. infusion set is 60 gtts./mL.

CHAPTER 8: SOLUTIONS

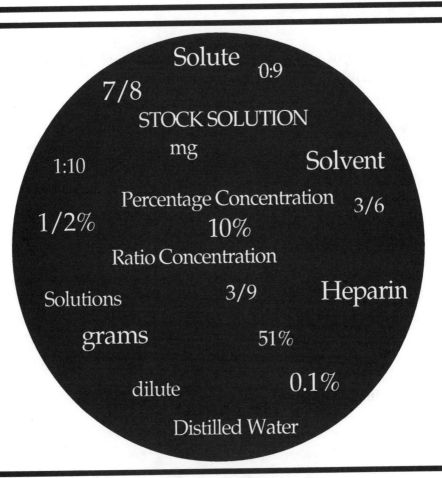

Solute 0:9

7/8

STOCK SOLUTION

mg

1:10

Solvent

Percentage Concentration 3/6

1/2% 10%

Ratio Concentration

Solutions 3/9 Heparin

grams 51%

dilute 0.1%

Distilled Water

CHAPTER 8

Objectives

1. The student will demonstrate an understanding of the terms *solution, solute, solvent,* and *stock solution.*

2. The student will demonstrate the ability to calculate the ratio concentration of a solution accurately.

3. The student will demonstrate the ability to calculate the percentage concentration of a solution accurately.

4. The student will demonstrate the ability to calculate the amount of solvent required to prepare a solution accurately.

5. The student will demonstrate the ability to dilute a stock solution accurately using the appropriate formula.

SOLUTIONS

A *solution* is a clear homogenous mixture that results from dissolving one or more substances in a liquid. There are two parts to a solution: the *solute* is the substance being dissolved, and the *solvent* is the liquid used in dissolving. The solvent generally used is distilled water. The concentration of a solution depends on the amount of solute used and the amount of solvent used. As a result, the concentration of a solution can be expressed as a percentage or ratio.

> *EXAMPLE:*   A 10% solution of dextrose means there are 10 parts of dextrose (drug) and approximately 90 parts of distilled water to make 100 parts of a solution.
>
> Written as a ratio, 10% dextrose = 10 : 100 = 1 : 10

Most solutions today are available ready for use, having been prepared by the manufacturer or a pharmacist. There are occasions when health professionals, such as nurses, may have to prepare or dilute a solution. It is important for these health professionals to be able to calculate the concentration of solutions. Remember that these calculations may involve percentages or ratios.

Labels on stock solutions may state the amount of drug that is dissolved in a given amount of solution, expressed as a percentage or ratio. Depending on how the physician orders the solution, the information on the label may have to be converted to ensure that the appropriate solution is used.

To CALCULATE the RATIO CONCENTRATION of a solution:

Express the drug and solvent as a ratio.

Remember:

A. Convert a fraction or decimal fraction to a whole number.

B. Express a percentage as a ratio.

C. Reduce to lowest terms.

EXAMPLE #1: What is the ratio concentration of 500 mL of a solution containing 10 mL of a pure drug?

Express the drug (10 mL) and the solvent (500 mL) as a ratio.

10 : 500

Reduce to lowest terms.

Ratio concentration = 1:50

EXAMPLE #2: What is the ratio concentration of 0.2% epinephrine?

Express a percentage as a ratio.
0.2% = 0.2 : 100

Convert a decimal fraction to a whole number.

0.2 : 100 =

2 : 1 000

Reduce to lowest terms.

2 : 1 000 =

Ratio concentration = 1 : 500

NOTE: See Appendix H for answers to questions in this chapter.

Calculate the ratio concentrations:

1.   10%

2.   1/2%

3.   56%

4.   25%

5.   7%

6. 109%

7. 65%

8. 2.5%

9. 82%

10. 51%

11. 3 g of a drug in 1 200 mL of distilled water.

12. 20 mg of a drug in 0.5 L of distilled water.

13. 0.5 g of a drug in 200 mL of distilled water.

14. 1 500 mL of distilled water containing 6 g of a drug.

15. 1 g of a drug in 500 mL distilled water.

16. 1.6 g of a drug in 1 400 mL of distilled water.

17. 0.1 mg of a drug in 1 L of distilled water.

18. 0.8 mg of a drug in 32 mL of distilled water.

19. 300 mL of distilled water containing 0.15 mg of a drug.

20. 15 g of a drug in 3 L of distilled water.

To CALCULATE the PERCENTAGE CONCENTRATION of a solution:

A formula is used to calculate the percentage concentration of a solution (Figure 8-1).

DRUG : SOLVENT : : PERCENT : 100

Figure 8-2: Formula for calculating percentage concentration.

EXAMPLE #1: What is the percentage concentration of a solution labelled 1 : 4?

DRUG : SOLVENT : : PERCENT : 100

$1 : 4 : : X : 100$

$4X = 100$

$X = {}^{100}/_4$

$X = 25\%$

Percentage concentration $= 25\%$

EXAMPLE #2: What is the percentage concentration of 3 g of a drug in 2 L of solution?

Before using the formula, convert 2 L to mL.

$2 L = 2\,000 \text{ mL}$

DRUG : SOLVENT : : PERCENT : 100

$3\,g : 2\,000\,mL : : X : 100$

$2\,000X = 300$

$X = {}^{300}/_{2\,000}$

$X = 0.15 \text{ or } 0.2\%$

Percentage concentration $= 0.2\%$

Calculate the percentage concentrations:

21. $1 : 7$

22. $2 : 9$

23. $7 : 14$

24. 1 : 100

25. 3/4

26. 1/15

27. 1/20

28. 5/12

29. 11/42

30. 6/10

31. 20 g of sorbitol powder in 100 mL of distilled water.

32. 0.40 g of a drug in 200 mL of distilled water.

33. 1 g of gentian violet in 100 mL of distilled water.

34. 4 g of boric acid in 250 mL of distilled water.

35. 8 mg of crystals in 50 mL of distilled water.

36. 125 mg of glucose in 2 L of distilled water.

37. 20 mg of a drug in 400 mL of distilled water.

38. 200 mL of distilled water containing 0.5 g of a drug.

39. 0.50 g of crystals in 25 mL of distilled water.

40. 300 g of salt in 600 mL of distilled water.

To CALCULATE the amount of SOLVENT required to prepare a solution:

The formula for calculating percentage concentration can be used to calculate the amount of solvent required to prepare a solution.

DRUG : SOLVENT : : PERCENT : 100

EXAMPLE: How much distilled water is required to make a 5% solution from 4 g of a drug?

> DRUG : SOLVENT : : PERCENT : 100

4 g : X : : 5 : 100

5X = 400

X = $^{400}/_5$

X = 80 mL

80 mL of distilled water is required to prepare a solution from 4 g of a drug.

Calculate the amount of solvent required:

41. 5% solution from 10 g of a drug.

42. 1/2% solution from 0.5 g of a drug.

43. 15% solution from 2 g of a drug.

44. 2% solution from 0.4 g of a drug.

45. 125% solution from 11 g of a drug.

46. 5% solution from 5 g of a drug.

47. 100% solution from 15 g of a drug.

48. 64% solution from 8 g of a drug.

49. 33% solution from 16 g of a drug.

50. 25% solution from 500 g of a drug.

DILUTING STOCK SOLUTIONS

When a pure drug is dissolved in a liquid, the result is a *stock solution*. A weaker solution can be made from a stock solution by diluting it with a solvent, such as distilled water. However, an order for a stronger solution requires preparation of a new solution.

To CALCULATE the amount of STOCK SOLUTION required to DILUTE:

A formula is used to calculate the amount of stock solution required to combine with a solvent to provide a weaker, dilute solution (Figure 8-2).

$$\frac{\text{Desired Strength}}{\text{Available Strength}} = \frac{\text{Amount to Use}}{\text{Amount to Make}}$$

Figure 8-2: Formula for diluting stock solutions.

The above formula can also be worked as a proportion (Figure 8-3).

Desired Strength : Available Strength : : Amt. to Use : Amt. to Make

Figure 8-3: Formula using proportions for diluting stock solutions.

EXAMPLE: Prepare 2 L of a 5% glucose solution from 75% stock solution of glucose.

METHOD #1

$$\frac{\text{Desired Strength}}{\text{Available Strength}} = \frac{\text{Amount to Use}}{\text{Amount to Make}}$$

$$\frac{5\%}{75\%} = \frac{X}{2\,L}$$

Cross-multiply:

$75X = 10$

$X = {}^{10}/_{75}$

$X = 0.133\,L$

METHOD #2

> Desired Str. : Avail. Str. : : Amt. to Use : Amt. to Make

$5\% : 75\% : : X : 2\,L$

$75X = 10$

$X = {}^{10}/_{75}$

$X = 0.133\,L$

0.133 L converted to mL = 133 mL

133 mL of 75% glucose stock solution is required.

2 L = 2 000 mL of 5% glucose solution is ordered.

2 000 mL - 133 mL = 1 867 mL

1 867 mL of solvent is combined with 133 mL of 75% glucose stock solution to provide 2 000 mL (2 L) of 5% glucose solution.

Calculate and state how to prepare the following solutions:

51. 1 L of 2% solution from a 50% stock solution.

52. 1 500 mL of 1% solution from a 20% stock solution.

53. 100 mL of 5% solution from a 25% stock solution.

54. 3 L of 10% solution from a 90% stock solution.

55. 500 mL of 60% solution from a 75% stock solution.

To CALCULATE the amount of SOLUTION that can be prepared from a KNOWN QUANTITY of a DRUG:

The formula for diluting stock solutions can be used to calculate the amount of solution that can be prepared from a known quantity of a drug.

$$\frac{\text{Desired Strength}}{\text{Available Strength}} = \frac{\text{Amount to Use}}{\text{Amount to Make}}$$

A drug may be a stock solution or a pure drug. A pure drug is 100 parts of the drug.

EXAMPLE: How much 5% solution can be prepared from 20 mL of a pure drug?

$$\frac{\text{Desired Strength}}{\text{Available Strength}} = \frac{\text{Amount to Use}}{\text{Amount to Make}}$$

$$\frac{5\%}{100\%} = \frac{20\text{ mL}}{X}$$

$5X = 2\,000$

$X = {}^{2\,000}/5$

$X = 400\text{ mL}$

400 mL of 5% solution can be prepared from 20 mL of a pure drug.

Calculate the amount of solution that can be prepared:

56. How much 10% solution can be prepared from 10 mL of a pure drug?

57. How much 25% solution can be prepared from 5 mL of a pure drug?

58. How much 50% solution can be prepared from 25 mL of a pure drug?

59. How much 20% solution can be prepared from 5 mL of a pure drug?

60. How much 1/4% solution can be prepared from 5 mL of a pure drug?

CHAPTER 9: POST-TEST

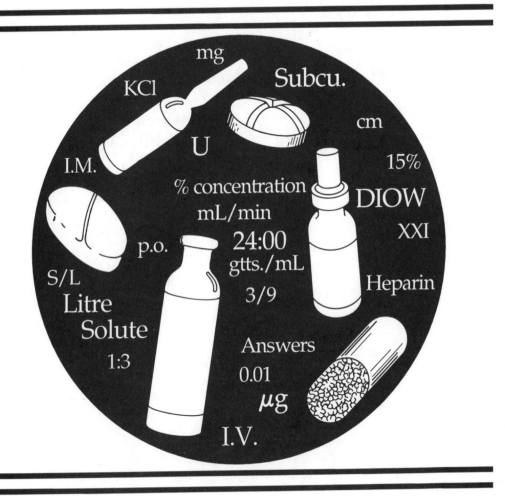

CHAPTER 9

Objectives

1. The student will demonstrate accuracy in completion of the practical examples provided.

2. The student will demonstrate improved performance in areas relevant to identified weaknesses.

Answer the following questions. Show any work needed to achieve the final answer. See Appendix I for answers to questions 1 through 200. Reduce to lowest terms where possible.

Convert to Roman numerals:

1. 9

2. 27

Convert to Arabic numerals:

3. XV$\overline{ss}$

4. XIX

Convert to whole or mixed numbers:

5. $24/6$

6. $17/3$

Convert to improper fractions:

7. $1 1/9$

8. $10 2/5$

Convert to whole numbers, proper fractions, or improper fractions:

9. $\dfrac{1/5}{1/2}$

10. $\dfrac{11/12}{4}$

Solve the following:

11. $6/7 + 1/9$

12. $7 1/8 + 3 1/3$

13. $7/11 - 1/4$

14. $4 1/12 - 1 5/6$

15. $22/10 \times 4/7$

16. $3 1/3 \times 9 1/8$

17. $17/18 \div 1/9$

18. $16 2/3 \div 4 1/3$

Convert to decimal fractions:

19. $2 1/10$

20. $7/11$

Convert to improper fractions:

21. 0.57

22. 0.6

Solve the following:

23.	0.471 + 1.92	24.	10.004 + 21.6
25.	7.327 - 0.909	26.	10.1 - 9.427
27.	0.018 x 0.179	28.	5.62 x 3.99
29.	9.03 ÷ 1.7	30.	116.34 ÷ 11.29
31.	0.005 x 10	32.	0.347 x 0.01
33.	350.91 ÷ 100	34.	5.594 ÷ 0.001

Convert to common fractions:

35. 67%　　　　　36. 9.5%

Convert to decimal fractions:

37. 92%　　　　　38. 3.75%

Convert to percentages:

39. $9\,1/5$　　　　40. $7/11$

41. 0.57　　　　　42. 5.32

Convert to ratios:

43. $3/4$　　　　　44. $50/250$

45. 0.65　　　　　46. 0.049

Convert to fractions:

47. 3 : 48　　　　48　11 : 12

Convert to decimal fractions:

49. 21 : 42　　　　50. 16 : 51

Convert to ratios:

51. 97%　　　　　52. 50%

Convert to percentages:

53. 4 : 11　　　　54. 9 : 54

Solve for X:

55. 9 : 24 : : X : 36　　　56. $1/2$: 8 : : X : 16

Convert the following:

57.	2.8 g	=	_____ mg	58.	0.33 L	=	_____ mL	
59.	1.1 g	=	_____ µg	60.	2.8 m	=	_____ cm	
61.	6 mol	=	_____ mmol	62.	5 mg	=	_____ g	
63.	16 mL	=	_____ L	64.	200 g	=	_____ kg	
65.	29 mm	=	_____ cm	66.	75 mcg	=	_____ mg	

Read the following questions carefully, and state whether they are correct or incorrect. State the correct answer where applicable.

67.	2.5 kg = 2 500 g.	68.	1 mL = 0.001 Litres
69.	1 m = 100 cms	70.	.1 g = 100 mg
71.	1 L = 1 000 mL	72.	100 g = 100,000 mg

Convert to 24-hour time:

73.	12:45 p.m.	74.	9:26 a.m.
75.	8:15 p.m.	76.	12:01 a.m.

Write the dates in metric:

77.	March 15, 1988	78.	April 3, 1988
79.	October 22, 1919	80.	December 18, 1955

Calculate the number of tablets or capsules administered for each dose and for a 24-hour period:

81. Metronidazole (Flagyl) 1 g p.o. stat. and 500 mg p.o. b.i.d. for three days. The medication is available in 500-mg capsules.

82. Diazepam (Valium) 3 mg p.o. h.s. p.r.n. The medication is available in 2-mg tablets scored in half.

83. Captopril (Capoten) 12.5 mg p.o. b.i.d. The medication is available in 25-mg tablets scored in half.

84. Diltiazem HCl (Cardizem) 90 mg p.o. q.i.d. The medication is available in 60-mg tablets scored in half.

85. Triazolam (Halcion) 0.5 mg p.o. h.s. The medication is available in 0.25-mg tablets scored in half.

86. Diphenhydramine HCl (Benadryl) 50 mg p.o. t.i.d. The medication is available in 25-mg capsules.

87. Prazosin HCl (Minipress) 0.5 mg p.o. t.i.d. The medication is available in 1-mg tablets scored in half.

88. Ampicillin sodium (Ampicin) 1 g p.o. stat. then 500 mg p.o. q.6h for 5 days. The medication is available in 500-mg capsules.

89. Clonidine HCl (Catapres) 0.1 mg p.o. b.i.d. The medication is available in 200-μg tablets scored in half.

90. Isorbide dinitrate (Isordil) 10 mg S/L stat. The medication is available in 5-mg tablets.

Calculate the amount of liquid administered for each dose and for a 24-hour period:

91. Digoxin (Lanoxin) elixir 0.5 mg p.o. o.d. The medication is available in 50 μg per mL.

92. Guaifenesin (Robitussin) syrup 75 mg p.o. q.4h. The medication is available in 100 mg per 5 mL.

93. Acetaminophen (Tylenol) elixir 150 mg p.o. t.i.d. The medication is available in 24 mg per mL.

94. Dimenhydrinate (Gravol) liquid 30 mg p.o. stat. The medication is available in 15 mg per 5 mL.

95. Nystatin (Mycostatin) suspension 100 000 U p.o. q.4h. The medication is available in 100 000 U per mL.

96. Potassium chloride (Kay Ciel) elixir 40 mEq p.o. o.d. The medication is available in 20 mmol per 15 mL.

97. Cephalexin (Keflex) suspension 250 mg p.o. q.6h. The medication is available in 125 mg per 5 mL.

98.   Docusate sodium (Colace) syrup 100 mg p.o. b.i.d. The medication is available in 20 mg per 5 mL.

99.   Diazepam (Valium) suspension 2.5 mg p.o. t.i.d. The medication is available in 5 mg per 5 mL.

100.   Thioridazine HCl (Mellaril) suspension 25 mg p.o. t.i.d. The medication is available in 10 mg per 5 mL.

Calculate the child's dose and the amount to administer for each dose and for a 24-hour period:

The CPS states a child's dose of :

101.   Theophylline (Theolair) liquid is 5 mg/kg q.8h. Theophylline liquid is available in 15 mL = 80 mg. The child weighs 18 kg.

102.   Acetaminophen (Tylenol) drops is 10 mg/kg q.6h. Acetaminophen drops are available in 0.8 mL = 80 mg. The child weighs 8 kg.

103.   Phenytoin (Dilantin) infatabs is 5 mg/kg/day in equal doses q.8h. Phenytoin infatabs are available in 50-mg tablets scored in half. The child weighs 15 kg.

104.   Cephalexin monohydrate (Keflex) suspension is 25 mg/kg q.6h. Cephalexin monohydrate suspension is available in 5 mL = 125 mg. The child weighs 10 kg.

105.   Ampicillin sodium (Ampicin) is 50 mg/kg/day in equal doses q.6h. Ampicillin sodium is available in 5 mL = 250 mg. The child weighs 16 kg.

Calculate the number of mL administered for each dose and for a 24-hour period:

106.   Phenobarbital sodium (Luminal) 120 mg I.M. q.6h p.r.n. The medication is available in 1-mL ampules containing 120 mg/mL.

107.   Prochlorperazine (Stemetil) 5 mg I.M. q.8h. The medication is available in 2-mL ampules containing 10 mg.

108.   Bethanechol chloride (Urecholine) 2.5 mg subcu. stat. The medication is available in 1-mL ampules containing 5 mg.

109.   Clindamycin phosphate (Dalacin C Phosphate) 300 mg I.V. t.i.d. The medication is available in 4-mL ampules containing 150 mg per mL.

110.   Naloxone HCl (Narcan) 100 µg I.V. stat. The medication is available in 1-mL ampules containing 400 µg.

111.   Dexamethasone sodium phosphate injection (Hexadrol Phosphate Injection) 10 mg I.V. stat. then 4 mg I.V. q.6h. The medication is available in 5-mL vials labelled 4 mg = 1 mL.

112.   Gentamicin sulfate (Garamycin) 100 mg I.V. q.8h. The medication is available in 2-mL multiple-dose vials labelled 1 mL = 40 mg.

113.   Chlorpromazine HCl (Largactil) 25 mg I.M. t.i.d. The medication is available in 2-mL ampules containing 50 mg.

114.   Ranitidine HCl (Zantac) 50 mg I.V. q.12h. The medication is available in 2-mL ampules containing 50 mg.

115.   Iron dextran complex (Imferon) 100 mg I.M. weekly. The medication is available in 2-mL ampules containing 50 mg/mL.

116.   Metoclopramide HCl (Reglan) 10 mg I.V. q.6h p.r.n. The medication is available in 2-mL ampules containing 5 mg/mL.

117. Benztropine mesylate (Cogentin) 2 mg I.M. q.12h p.r.n. The medication is available in 2-mL ampules containing 2 mg.

118. Vitamin B_{12} (Rubramin) 100 µg I.M. monthly. The medication is available in 10-mL vials containing 1 000 µg/mL.

119. Cloxacillin sodium monohydrate (Orbenin) 0.25 g I.V. q.6h. The medication is available in a 500-mg vial. Instructions are to add 1.7 mL of sterile water to yield 2 mL.

120. Penicillin G sodium (Crystapen) 500 000 U I.V. q.6h. The medication is available in a 1 000 000-U vial. The dilution table on the label reads:

Potency required I.U. per mL	Add sterile aqueous diluent
200 000	4.6 mL
250 000	3.6 mL
500 000	1.6 mL
750 000	0.9 mL

121. Cloxacillin sodium (Tegopen) 250 mg I.V. q.6h. The medication is available in a 2 000-mg vial. Instructions are to add 20 mL of sterile water to yield a solution containing 100 mg/mL.

122. Cefoxitin sodium (Mefoxin) 1 g I.V. q.6h. The medication is available in a 1-g vial. Instructions are to add 10 mL of sterile water to yield 10.5 mL, providing a solution containing 95 mg/mL.

123. Conjugated estrogens (Premarin) 25 mg I.M. stat. The medication is available in a 25-mg vial. Instructions are to add 5 mL of sterile water.

Calculate the child's dose and the number of mL to administer for each dose and for a 24-hour period:

The CPS states a child's dose of:

124. Pancuronium bromide (Pavulon) is 100 g/kg. The medication is available in 5-mL ampules containing 1 mg per mL. The child weighs 9 kg.

125. Phenytoin (Dilantin) is initially 5 mg/kg/day in equally divided doses q.8h. The medication is available in 2-mL ampules containing 50 mg/mL. The child weighs 12 kg.

126. Chlorpromazine HCl (Largactil) is 0.5 mg/kg. The medication is available in a 2-mL ampule containing 50 mg. The child weighs 25 kg.

127. Gentamicin (Cidomycin) is 3 mg/kg/day in equal doses q.8h. The medication is available in 2-mL multiple-dose pediatric vials containing 10 mg/mL. The child weighs 21 kg.

128. Naloxone HCl (Narcan) is 10 µg/kg. The medication is available in 1-mL ampules containing 0.4 mg. The child weighs 4 kg.

Calculate the number of mL to be administered for each dose (each insulin is supplied in 10-mL vials labelled 1 mL = 100 U):

129. Humulin-R 10 units and Humulin-N 22 units subcu. a.c. q.a.m.

130. Initard Human insulin 25 U subcu. @ 07:30 and @ 16:30 o.d.

131. Velosulin 8 units S.C. stat.

132. Insulatard insulin 29 units subcu. a.c. q.a.m.

133. P.Z.I. 15 U subcu. a.c. q.a.m.

134. Novolin-30/70 insulin 30 units S.C. 45 min a.c. q.a.m.

135. Lente insulin 56 units and Toronto insulin 10 units
      a.c. q.a.m.

136. Novolin-Lente insulin 15 units subcu. a.c. q.a.m.

137. NPH insulin 25 units and Toronto insulin 10 units
      subcu. a.c. q.a.m.

138. Novolin-Toronto insulin 10 units subcu. stat.

139. Heparin 8 000 U subcu. q.8h. The medication is
      available in a 10-mL vial labelled 1 mL = 10 000 U.

140. Heparin 3 000 U subcu. b.i.d. The medication is
      available in a 5-mL vial labelled 1 mL = 10 000 U.

141. Heparin 10 000 U I.V. q 6h. The medication is
      available in a 10-mL vial labelled 1 mL = 1 000 U.

142. Heparin 4 000 U I.V. push. The medication is
      available in a 10-mL vial labelled 1 mL = 1 000 U.

143. Heparin 5 000 U subcu. q.8h. The medication is
      available in a 5-mL vial labelled 1 mL = 10 000 U.

Calculate the amount of I.V. additive required:

144. Potassium chloride 40 mmol/L. Prepare 1 000 mL of
      I.V. $^2/_3$ & $^1/_3$ Potassium chloride is available in a
      10-mL single-dose vial labelled 20 mmol.

145. Potassium chloride 30 mmol/L. Prepare 1 L of I.V.
      N/S. Potassium chloride is available in a 20-mL
      multiple-dose vial labelled 40 mmol.

146. KCl 15 mEq/500 mL I.V. Prepare I.V. R/L 500 mL. KCl
      is available in a 10-mL ampule containing 20 mmol.

147. Toronto insulin 20 U in 1 000 mL I.V. D5W. Toronto
      insulin is available in a 10-mL multiple-dose vial
      labelled 1 mL = 100 U.

148.   MgSO$_4$ 2 g in 500 mL I.V. D5W @ 175 mL/h o.d.
         MgSO$_4$ is available in a 10-mL ampule containing 5 g.

149.   Heparin 900 U I.V. q.1h. Infuse I.V. N/S 500 mL @
         50 mL/h. The medication is available in a 10-mL vial
         labelled 1 mL = 1 000 U.

150.   Heparin 650 U I.V. q.1h. Infuse I.V. N/S 500 mL @
         50 mL/h. The medication is available in a 5-mL vial
         labelled 1 mL = 1 000 U.

151.   Heparin 500 U I.V. q.1h. Infuse I.V. N/S 500 mL @
         50 mL/h. The medication is available in a 10-mL vial
         labelled 1 mL = 1 000 U.

152.   Heparin 800 U I.V. q.1h. Infuse I.V. $^2/_3$ & $^1/_3$ 500 mL @
         50 mL/h. The medication is available in a 10-mL vial
         labelled 1 mL = 1 000 U.

153.   Heparin 550 U I.V. q.1h. Infuse I.V. $^2/_3$ & $^1/_3$ 500 mL @
         50 mL/h.The medication is available in a 10-mL vial
         labelled 1 mL = 1 000 U.

154.   Aminophylline 45 mg/h in I.V. N/S 500 mL @
         45 mL/h. The medication is available in a 10-mL
         ampule containing 500 mg.

155.   Aminophylline 35 mg/h in I.V. D5W 500 mL @
         35 mL/h. The medication is available in a 10-mL
         ampule containing 500 mg.

Calculate the flow rates using the general formula:

156.   I.V. D5W @ 100 mL/h. The I.V. infusion set delivers 10 gtts./mL.

157.   I.V. $2/3$ & $1/3$ @ 125 mL/h. The I.V. infusion set delivers 10 gtts./mL.

158.   I.V. Ringer's lactate solution @ 75 mL/h x 1 hour, then increase to 150 mL/h. The I.V. infusion set delivers 10 gtts./mL.

159.   I.V. N/S @ 175 mL/h. The I.V. infusion set delivers 60 gtts./mL.

160.   I.V. D5W @ 40 mL/h. The I.V. infusion set delivers 60 gtts./mL.

Calculate the flow rates using the metric standard formula:

161.   I.V. 5% D/S @ 3 mL/min. The drop factor for the I.V. infusion set is 10 gtts./mL.

162.   I.V. $2/3$ & $1/3$ @ 3.3 mL/min x 1 hour, then decrease to 1.5 mL/min. The drop factor for the I.V. infusion set is 10 gtts./mL.

163.   I.V. 0.9% sodium chloride @ 2.5 mL/min. The drop factor for the I.V. infusion set is 60 gtts./mL.

164.   I.V. normal saline @ 0.5 mL/min. The drop factor for the I.V. infusion set is 15 gtts./mL.

165.   I.V. D10W @ 1.5 mL/min. The drop factor for the I.V. infusion set is 20 gtts./mL.

Calculate the flow rates using the general formula:

166.   1 000 mL of I.V. 10% dextrose & water over 5 hours. The drop factor for the I.V. infusion set is 10 gtts./mL.

167.   600 mL of I.V. R/L over 5 hours. The drop factor for the I.V. infusion set is 10 gtts./mL.

168. I.V. N/S 400 mL over 2 hours, then 1 000 mL over 8 hours. The drop factor for the I.V. infusion set is 60 gtts./mL.

169. 280 mL of I.V. $^2/_3$ & $^1/_3$ over 4 hours. The drop factor for the I.V. infusion set is 60 gtts./mL.

170. I.V. R/L 360 mL over 3 hours, then 3 000 mL over 20 hours. The drop factor for the I.V. infusion set is 20 gtts./mL.

Calculate the flow rates using the metric standard formula:

171. 0.9% sodium chloride 1 000 mL over 10 hours. The drop factor for the I.V. infusion set is 60 gtts./mL.

172. I.V. D10W 500 mL over 4 hours. The drop factor for the I.V. infusion set is 10 gtts./mL.

173. 2 500 mL of I.V. $^2/_3$ & $^1/_3$ over 20 hours. The drop factor for the I.V. infusion set is 20 gtts./mL.

174. 3 000 mL of I.V. Ringer's lactate solution over 24 hours, then 1 000 mL of I.V. 5% dextrose and saline over 10 hours. The drop factor for the I.V. infusion set is 10 gtts./mL.

175. 50 mL of I.V. N/S over 20 minutes, then 1 000 mL of I.V. $^2/_3$ & $^1/_3$ over 5 hours. The drop factor for the I.V. infusion set is 60 gtts./mL.

Calculate the ratio concentrations:

176. 8%

177. 15%

178. 75%

179. 27%

180. $^1/_4$%

Calculate the percentage concentrations:

181.   1 : 8

182.   9 : 15

183. $^7/_{16}$

184. $^4/_9$

185.   1 g of gentian violet in 225 mL of distilled water.

Calculate the amount of solvent required:

186.   25% solution from 1 g of a drug.

187.   10% solution from 5 g of a drug.

188. $^1/_2$% solution from 1 g of a drug.

189.   50% solution from 5 g of a drug.

190.   20% solution from 2 g of a drug.

Calculate and state how to prepare:

191.   125 mL of 5% solution from a 10% stock solution.

192.   500 mL of 25% solution from a 30% stock solution.

193.   300 mL of 40% solution from a 90% stock solution.

194.   1 L of 10% solution from a 20% stock solution.

195.   1 500 mL of 15% solution from a 75% stock solution.

Calculate the amount of solution that can be prepared:

196.   How much 2% solution can be prepared from 10 mL of a pure drug?

197.   How much 10% solution can be prepared from 5 mL of a pure drug?

198.   How much 20% solution can be prepared from 200 mL of a pure drug?

199.   How much 25% solution can be prepared from 20 mL of a pure drug?

200.   How much $1/2$% solution can be prepared from 15 mL of a pure drug?

APPENDICES

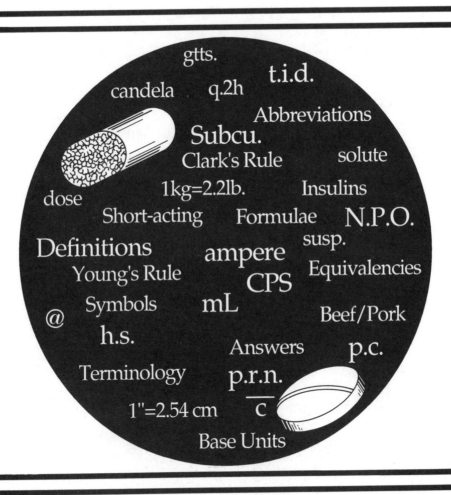

gtts.

t.i.d.

candela   q.2h

Abbreviations

Subcu.

Clark's Rule   solute

dose   1kg=2.2lb.   Insulins

Short-acting   Formulae   N.P.O.

susp.

Definitions   ampere

Young's Rule   Equivalencies

CPS

@   Symbols   mL   Beef/Pork

h.s.

Answers   p.c.

Terminology   p.r.n.

1"=2.54 cm   c̄

Base Units

APPENDIX A

Answers to Chapter 1: Pretest

1.	viii (VIII)	24.	$2/15$	47.	$129/200$
2.	xiv (XIV)	25.	$2\,23/27$	48.	$18/25$
3.	xvi (XVI)	26.	$1\,11/21$	49.	0.373 6
4.	xxv (XXV)	27.	$1/12$	50.	10.452
5.	12	28.	$5/33$	51.	0.244
6.	17	29.	$7/12$	52.	6.171 2
7.	15	30.	$9/25$	53.	0.628
8.	24	31.	$8\,1/8$	54.	1.995 82
9.	$2\,1/3$	32.	$2\,3/16$	55.	0.007 11
10.	1	33.	$1/14$	56.	17.209
11.	$15/7$	34.	$3/35$	57.	0.05
12.	$13/4$	35.	$4\,3/8$	58.	0.073
13.	$2/66$	36.	$1\,1/6$	59.	0.008
14.	$63/3$	37.	$1\,6/7$	60.	29.32
15.	$7/11$	38.	$2\,3/13$	61.	100.455 9
16.	$3/5$	39.	$2\,4/19$	62.	0.561 7
17.	$1\,1/4$	40.	$2\,18/65$	63.	765
18.	$1\,17/28$	41.	0.200	64.	27 340
19.	$5\,1/2$	42.	0.003	65.	35.86
20.	$7\,3/40$	43.	0.240	66.	102.97
21.	$1/7$	44.	0.167	67.	1.017
22.	$5/19$	45.	$4/25$	68.	4 000
23.	$1/3$	46.	$3/10$	69.	$1/500$

70.	$33/100$	81.	$1/10$	92.	X = 150
71.	0.1	82.	$1/12$	93.	Numerator
72.	0.008	83.	0.857	94.	Denominator
73.	20%	84.	3.444	95.	$27\,8/100$
74.	1%	85.	1 : 4	96.	Improper fraction
75.	60%	86.	57 : 100		
76.	208%	87.	25%	97.	Lowest common denominator
77.	5 : 9	88.	36%		
78.	2 : 3	89.	X = 40	98.	0.05
79.	113 : 200	90.	X = $8/15$	99.	19 : 57
80.	2 : 5	91.	X = 0.004	100.	11 : 2 : : 33 : 6

APPENDIX B

Answers to Chapter 2: Arithmetic Review   Pages 12–39

1.	II or ii	23.	$9/5$	46.	$1\,2/7$
2.	IX$\overline{\overline{SS}}$ or IX$\overline{\overline{SS}}$	24.	$153/70$	47.	$5\,1/2$
	ixss or ixss	25.	112	48.	$2\,23/160$
3.	XIII or xiii	26.	$1/2$	49.	$25\,13/15$
4.	LIX or lix	27.	$1/4$	50.	$14\,2/3$
5.	XXI or xxi	28.	24	51.	0.125
6.	12	29.	$6\,9/29$	52.	0.467
7.	45	30.	$3\,5/19$	53.	0.333
8.	55	31.	$3/7$	54.	5.200
9.	114	32.	$19/20$	55.	11.333
10.	$30\,1/2$	33.	$9\,1/2$	56	$371/500$
11.	1	34.	$22\,5/18$	57.	$7/100$
12.	11	35.	$36\,5/66$	58.	$23/50$
13.	$1\,3/5$	36.	$7/12$	59.	$19/100$
14.	$8\,1/11$	37.	$19/30$	60.	$9/10$
15.	$2\,13/15$	38.	$1\,27/70$	61.	4.109
16.	$22/7$	39.	$4\,2/35$	62.	0.048 3
17.	$17/8$	40.	$3\,17/20$	63.	0.047
18.	$23/2$	41.	$14/15$	64.	72.041 4
19.	$43/6$	42.	$6/187$	65.	667.51
20.	$32/6$	43.	$31\,8/9$	66.	0.005 27
21.	$1/4$	44.	$18\,3/4$	67.	0.749
22.	$1/84$	45.	$86\,1/39$	68.	9.288

69.	493.988	99.	78 333	129.	1 750.1
70.	3.420 1	100.	4 670 3	130.	1 303.1
71.	0.556 6	101.	0.023 04	131.	$1/200$
72.	56.959	102.	0.002 9	132.	$3/20$
73.	21.426 6	103.	0.015 623	133.	$7/25$
74.	309.721 7	104.	0.369 2	134.	$13/400$
75.	0.000 012 18	105.	0.000 001	135.	$53/100$
76.	192.697 9	106.	10.667	136.	0.18
77.	1 701.564 326 4	107.	0.420 07	137.	0.9
78.	6.394	108.	37.704 7	138.	0.075
79.	27.667 5	109.	0.010 891	139.	0.72
80.	314.215 968	110.	16.324 1	140.	0.08
81.	5.469	111.	0.001	141.	14.29%
82.	504	112.	0.106 2	142.	27.27%
83.	4.038	113.	0.156 34	143.	750%
84.	4.419	114.	0.000 000 36	144.	140%
85.	26.658	115.	1.719	145.	75%
86.	1.961	116.	1.516 1 1	146.	32%
87.	14.428	117.	0.369 9	147.	10.16%
88.	192.222	118.	0.004 603	148.	0.7%
89.	1.105	119.	0.000 71	149.	100.15%
90.	9.296	120.	1.892 1	150.	1 604%
91.	3.2	121.	4.2	151.	1 : 8
92.	27.14	122.	1 026	152.	11 : 12
93.	4.7	123.	3 140	153.	1 : 2
94.	17 321	124.	1 426 700	154.	9 : 17
95.	1 276.9	125.	30	155.	1 : 5
96.	6 888	126.	8 906	156.	1 : 10
97.	104.9	127.	111 200	157.	43 : 200
98.	100 104	128.	10.2	158.	1 603 : 10 000

159. 3 971 : 5 000

160. 13 : 2 500

161. $^1/_5$

162. $^{16}/_{39}$

163. $^{14}/_{53}$

164. $^{10}/_{101}$

165. $^7/_{13}$

166. 0.714

167. 0.2

168. 0.387

169. 0.439

170. 0.059

171. 3 : 25

172. 3 : 5

173. 73 : 100

174. 17 : 100

175. 2 : 25

176. 12.5%

177. 42.86%

178. 45.83%

179. 22.22%

180. 34.04%

181. X = 2

182. X = 26.667 or
     X = 26 $^2/_3$

183. X = 8

184. X = 3

185. X = 60

186. X = 60.784 or
     X = 60 $^{40}/_{51}$

187. X = 4.167 or
     X = 4 $^1/_6$

188. X = 1

189. X = 64

190. X = 2.92 or
     X = 2 $^{11}/_{12}$

191. X = 0.15 or
     X = $^3/_{20}$

192. X = 0.133 or
     X = $^2/_{15}$

193. X = 0.312 5 or
     X = 0.313 or
     X = $^5/_{16}$

194. X = 500

195. X = 0.6

196. X = 0.333

197. X = 1.1

198. X = 2

199. X = 32

200. X = 4

APPENDIX C

Answers to Chapter 3: Metric System   Pages 45–60

1.	Apothecary, household	25.	5 000 mmol
2.	Base units	26.	300 g
3.	10	27.	1 800 g
4.	Litre	28.	950 mL
5.	kilo	29.	300 000 mg
6.	g	30.	70 mm
7.	mL	31.	2 100 mL
8.	L	32.	15 000 mg
9.	mg	33.	1 900 g
10.	kg	34.	8 500 mL
11.	nmol	35.	2 300 mL
12.	cm	36.	5 100 mL
13.	m	37.	90 000 mg
14.	k	38.	115 000 mg
15.	m	39.	7 500 mm
16.	3 000 g	40.	3 200 mmol
17.	250 mL	41.	850 000 mg
18.	100 mL	42.	120 000 mcm
19.	5 300 mg	43.	8 000 mmol
20.	100 000 mcg	44.	3 000 000 mg
21.	750 mg	45.	100 dL
22.	10 000 µg	46.	1 100 mL
23.	2 000 000 000 mcg	47.	25 mL
24.	1 000 000 mg	48.	150 mm

49.	150 cm		77.	0.001 050 kg or 0.001 05 kg	
50.	1 500 mm		78.	1.16 m	
51.	0.400 g or 0.4 g		79.	0.000 09 cm	
52.	0.610 L or 0.61 L		80.	0.000 75 mm	
53.	1.010 g or 1.01 g		81.	10 cm	
54.	0.090 mg or 0.09 mg		82.	4.5 cm	
55.	0.450 kg or 0.45 kg		83.	0.000 306 m	
56.	0.095 L		84.	0.97 m	
57.	5 g		85.	0.002 1 m	
58.	0.250 L or 0.25 L		86.	Incorrect	15 g
59.	0.115 L		87.	Incorrect	96 g
60.	365.0 L or 365 L		88.	Incorrect	0.6 L
61.	1.520 kg or 1.52 kg		89.	Incorrect	0.49 g
62.	0.68 dL		90.	Correct	
63.	1.58 dL		91.	Incorrect	10°C
64.	0.450 L or 0.45 L		92.	Incorrect	30 g or thirty grams
65.	2.350 L or 2.35 L				
66.	0.325 g		93.	Correct	
67.	0.4 cm		94.	Incorrect	1 g
68.	0.016 mol		95.	Incorrect	1 000 mL
69.	0.025 mol		96.	Correct	
70.	0.000 5 mol		97.	Incorrect	0.5 mmol
71.	0.5 L		98.	Incorrect	2.3 L
72.	1.500 kg or 1.5 kg		99.	Incorrect	7 μg
73.	0.000 05 mg		100.	Correct	
74.	2.50 L or 2.5 L		101.	07:35	
75.	0.000 000 500 kg or 0.000 000 5 kg		102.	12:00	
			103.	10:23	
76.	0.000 360 kg or 0.000 36 kg		104.	17:30	
			105.	23:00	

106. 02:53
107. 19:35
108. 00:00 or 24:00
109. 00:05
110. 21:17

111. 89/01/01 or 89-01-01
112. 82/07/03 or 82-07-03
113. 77/07/08 or 77-07-08
114. 85/03/28 or 85-03-28
115. 54/09/09 or 54-09-09

APPENDIX D

Answers to Chapter 4: Oral Dosages

Tablets and Capsules   Page 73

1. 2 tablets x 2 times a day = 4 tablets in 24 hours

2. 1 tablet x 4 times a day = 4 tablets in 24 hours

3. 8 tablets at bedtime

4. 0.25 tablet x 3 times a day = 0.75 tablet in 24 hours

5. 2 tablets at bedtime

6. 0.5 tablet at bedtime

7. 2 capsules x 2 times a day = 4 capsules in 24 hours

8. 2 capsules x 2 times a day = 4 capsules in 24 hours

9. 2 capsules at bedtime if necessary

10. 1 tablet x 3 times a day and 4 tablets at bedtime = 7 tablets in 24 hours

Liquids   Pages 77–78

11. 12.5 mL x 4 times a day = 50 mL in 24 hours

12. 2 mL x 4 times a day = 8 mL in 24 hours

13. 2.5 mL once a day

14. 7.5 mL x 3 times a day = 22.5 mL in 24 hours

15. 10 mL x 2 times a day = 20 mL in 24 hours

16. 12.5 mL x 3 times a day = 37.5 mL in 24 hours

17. 12.5 mL x 4 times a day = 50 mL in 24 hours

18. 10 mL x 6 times a day = 60 mL in 24 hours

19. 37.5 mL x 4 times a day = 150 mL in 24 hours

20. 50 mL once a day

Children's   Page 80–81

21. 1 000 mg = child's dose. Each 250-mg dose = 5 mL x 4
     times a day = 20 mL in 24 hours

22. 20 mg = child's dose. Each 10-mg dose = 1 mL x 2 times a
     day = 2 mL in 24 hours

23. 600 mg = child's dose. Each 150-mg dose = 6 mL x 4
     times a day = 24 mL in 24 hours

24. 85 mg = child's dose. Each 42.5-mg dose = 7.08 or 7.1 mL
     x 2 times a day = 14.2 mL in 24 hours

25. 90 mg = child's dose. Each 22.5-mg dose = 0.23 mL x 4
     times a day = 0.92 mL in 24 hours

APPENDIX E

Answers to Chapter 5: Parenteral Dosages   Pages 92–101

Ampules and Vials   Page 92

1. 0.5 mL x 4 times a day = 2 mL in 24 hours if necessary

2. 0.5 mL immediately

3. 0.5 mL x 6 times a day = 3 mL in 24 hours if necessary

4. 3.0 mL once a day

5. 5 mL immediatel

6. 0.5 mL x 4 times a day = 2 mL in 24 hours if necessary

7. 1 mL 45 minutes before surgery

8. 2 mL x 4 times a day = 8 mL in 24 hours

9. 1 mL at bedtime if necessary

10. 0.5 mL once a day

Reconstituted Medications   Page 98

11. 2 mL x 4 times a day = 8 mL in 24 hours

12. 2.2 mL x 2 doses = 4.4 mL

13. 4 mL immediately

14. 2 mL x 4 times a day = 8 mL in 24 hours

15. 1 mL x 6 times a day = 6 mL in 24 hours

Children's   Pages 100–101

16. 4 mg = child's dose = 0.8 mL

17. 36 mg = child's dose. Each 12-mg dose = 0.3 mL x 3 times
     a day = 0.9 mL in 24 hours

18. 960 μg = 0.96 mg = child's dose = 0.48 mL = 0.5 mL

19. 0.3 mg = child's dose = 2.4 mL

20. 11 mg = child's dose = 0.22 = 0.2 mL x 6 times a day =
     1.2 mL in 24 hours

APPENDIX F

Answers to Chapter 6: Insulin, Heparin, and I.V. Additives

Insulin   Page 107

1. 0.4 mL
2. 0.35 mL @ 07:30
    0.1 mL @ 16:30
3. 0.12 mL
4. 0.1 mL
5. 0.35 mL NPH + 0.25 mL Toronto = 0.6 mL

Heparin   Page 109

6. 0.6 mL
7. 0.3 mL
8. 1 mL
9. 0.5 mL
10. 7 mL

I.V. Additives   Page 111-112

11. 3.75 mL = 3.8 mL
12. 0.15 mL
13. 10 mL
14. 0.25 mL
15. 5 mL

I.V. Heparin and Aminophylline   Page 117

16. Add 0.7 mL hourly or 7 mL to 500 mL I.V. N/S

17. Add 0.6 mL hourly or 6 mL to 500 mL I.V. N/S

18. Add 0.45 mL hourly or 4.5 mL to 500 mL I.V. N/S

19. Add 10 mL to 500 mL I.V. normal saline

20. Add 10 mL to 500 mL I.V. D5W

APPENDIX G

Answers to Chapter 7: Intravenous Flow Rates

Pages 123–127

1. 46.6 = 47 gtts./min
2. 100 gtts./min
3. 25 gtts./min
4. 66.6 = 67 gtts./min x 3 h, then 41.6 = 42 gtts./min
5. 75 gtts./min x 1 h, then 125 gtts./min

6. 40 gtts./min
7. 180 gtts./min
8. 26 gtts./min
9. 20 gtts./min
10. 150 gtts./min

11. 12.5 = 13 gtts./min
12. 25 gtts./min
13. 50 gtts./min
14. 31.3 = 32 gtts./min(blood), then 20.8 = 21 gtts./min (N/S)
15. R/L 75 gtts./min x 10 h, then D5W 100 gtts./min x 20 h

16. 25 gtts./min
17. 125 or 126 gtts./min
18. 66 or 67 gtts./min x 5 h, then 33 or 34 gtts./min x 10 h
19. 25 gtts./min x 20 min, then 21 gtts./min x 24 h
20. 198 or 200 gtts./min

APPENDIX H

Answers to Chapter 8: Solutions

Ratio Concentrations   Pages 132–133

1. 1 : 10	8. 1 : 40	15. 1 : 500
2. 1 : 200	9. 41 : 50	16. 1 : 875
3. 14 : 25	10. 51 : 100	17. 1 : 10 000
4. 1 : 4	11. 1 : 400	18. 1 : 40
5. 7 : 100	12. 1 : 25	19. 1 : 2 000
6. 109 : 100	13. 1 : 400	20. 1 : 200
7. 13 : 20	14. 1 : 250	

Percentage Concentrations   Pages 134–135

21. 14.3%	28. 41.6%	35. 16%
22. 22.2%	29. 26.2%	36. 6.25%
23. 50%	30. 60%	37. 5%
24. 1%	31. 20%	38. 0.25%
25. 75%	32. 0.2%	39. 2%
26. 6.66%	33. 1%	40. 50%
27. 5%	34. 1.6%	

Amount of Solvent Required   Page 136

41. 200 mL	45. 8.8 mL	49. 48.48 mL or
42. 100 mL	46. 100 mL	48.5 mL
43. 13.3 mL	47. 15 mL	50. 2 000 mL
44. 20 mL	48. 12.5 mL	

Diluting Stock Solutions Page 138

51.   960 mL of solvent is combined with 40 mL of 50% stock
       solution to provide 1 000 mL (1 L) of 2% solution.
       960 mL + 40 mL = 1 000 mL = 1 L

52.   1 425 mL of solvent is combined with 75 mL of 20% stock
       solution to provide 1 500 mL of 1% solution.
       1 425 mL + 75 mL = 1 500 mL

53.   80 mL of solvent is combined with 20 mL of 25% stock
       solution to provide 100 mL of 5% solution.
       80 mL + 20 mL = 100 mL

54.   2 666.7 mL of solvent is combined with 333.3 mL of 90%
       stock solution to provide 3 000 mL (3 L) of 10% solution.
       2 666.7 mL + 333.3 mL = 3 000 mL = 3L

55.   100 mL of solvent is combined with 400 mL of 75% stock
       solution to provide 500 mL of 60% solution.
       100 mL + 400 mL = 500 mL

Preparing Solution from Pure Drug Pages 139–140

56.   100 mL

57.   20 mL

58.   50 mL

59.   25 mL

60.   2 000 mL

APPENDIX I

Answers to Chapter 9: Post-test   Pages 143–156

1.	ix (IX)	25.	6.418
2.	xxvii (XXVII)	26.	0.673
3.	$15^1/_2$	27.	0.003 22
4.	19	28.	22.423 8
5.	4	29.	5.311 7
6.	$5^2/_3$	30.	10.304 6
7.	$^{10}/_9$	31.	0.05
8.	$^{52}/_5$	32.	0.003 47
9.	$^2/_5$	33.	3.509 1
10.	$^{11}/_{48}$	34.	5 594
11.	$^{61}/_{63}$	35.	$^{67}/_{100}$
12.	$10^{11}/_{24}$	36.	$^{19}/_{200}$
13.	$^{17}/_{44}$	37.	0.92
14.	$2^1/_4$	38.	0.037 5
15.	$^{19}/_{35}$	39.	920%
16.	$30^5/_{12}$	40.	63.63%
17.	$8^1/_2$	41.	57%
18.	$3^{51}/_{65}$	42.	532%
19.	2.1	43.	3 : 4
20.	0.636	44.	1 : 5
21.	$^{57}/_{100}$	45.	13 : 20
22.	$^2/_3$	46.	49 : 1 000
23.	2.391	47.	$^1/_{16}$
24.	31.604	48.	$^{11}/_{12}$

49. 0.5
50. 0.313 7
51. 97 : 100
52. 1 : 2
53. 36.36%
54. 16.66%
55. X = 13.5
56. X = 1
57. 2 800 mg
58. 330 mL
59. 1 100 000.0 µg
60. 280 cm
61. 6 000 mmol
62. 0.005 g
63. 0.016 L
64. 0.2 kg
65. 2.9 cm

66. 0.075 mg
67. Incorrect; 2.5 kg = 2 500 g
68. Incorrect; 1 mL = 0.001 L
69. Incorrect; 1 m = 100 cm
70. Incorrect; 0.1 g = 100 mg
71. Incorrect; 1 L = 1 000 mL
72. Incorrect; 100 g = 100 000 mg
73. 12:45
74. 09:26
75. 20:15
76. 00:01
77. 88/03/15 or 88-03-15
78. 88/04/03 or 88-04-03
79. 19/10/22 or 19-10-22
80. 55/12/18 or 55-12-18

81. 2 tablets immediately and 1 tablet x 2 times a day = 4 tablets in the first 24 hours, then 2 tablets in 24 hours

82. 1.5 tablets at bedtime if necessary

83. 0.5 tablet x 2 times a day = 1 tablet in 24 hours

84. 1.5 tablets x 4 times a day = 6 tablets in 24 hours

85. 2 tablets at bedtime

86. 2 capsules x 3 times a day = 6 capsules in 24 hours

87. 0.5 tablet x 3 times a day = 1.5 tablets in 24 hours

88. 2 capsules immediately and 1 capsule x 4 times a day = 6 capsules in the first 24 hours, then 4 capsules in 24 hours

89. 0.5 tablet x 2 times a day = 1 tablet in 24 hours

90. 2 tablets immediately

91. 10 mL once a day

92. 3.75 = 3.8 mL x 6 times a day = 22.8 mL in 24 hours

93. 6.25 = 6.3 mL x 3 times a day = 18.9 mL in 24 hours

94. 10 mL immediately

95. 1 mL x 6 times a day = 6 mL in 24 hours

96. 30 mL once a day

97. 10 mL x 4 times a day = 40 mL in 24 hours

98. 25 mL x 2 times a day = 50 mL in 24 hours

99. 2.5 mL x 3 times a day = 7.5 mL in 24 hours

100. 12.5 mL x 3 times a day = 37.5 mL in 24 hours

101. 90 mg = child's dose. Each 90-mg dose = 16.88 = 16.9 mL x 3 times a day = 50.7 mL in 24 hours

102. 80 mg = child's dose. Each 80-mg dose = 0.8 mL x 4 times a day = 3.2 mL in 24 hours

103. 75 mg = child's dose. Each 25-mg dose = 0.5 tablet x 3 times a day = 1.5 tablets in 24 hours

104. 250 mg = child's dose. Each 250-mg dose = 10 mL x 4 times a day = 40 mL in 24 hours

105. 800 mg = child's dose. Each 200-mg dose = 4 mL x 4 times a day = 16 mL in 24 hours

106. 1 mL x 4 times a day = 4 mL in 24 hours if necessary

107. 1 mL x 3 times a day = 3 mL in 24 hours

108. 0.5 mL immediately

109. 2 mL x 3 times a day = 6 mL in 24 hours

110. 0.25 mL = 0.3 mL immediately

111. 2.5 mL immediately and 1 mL x 4 times a day = 6.5 mL in the first 24 hours, then 4 mL in 24 hours

112. 2.5 mL x 3 times a day = 7.5 mL in 24 hours

113. 1 mL x 3 times a day = 3 mL in 24 hours

114. 2 mL x 2 times a day = 4 mL

115. 2 mL weekly

116. 2 mL x 4 times a day = 8 mL in 24 hours if necessary

117. 2 mL x 2 times a day = 4 mL in 24 hours if necessary

118. 0.1 mL monthly

119. 1 mL x 4 times a day = 4 mL in 24 hours

120. 1 mL x 6 times a day = 6 mL in 24 hours

121. 2.5 mL x 4 times a day = 10 mL in 24 hours

122. 10.5 mL x 3 times a day = 31.5 mL in 24 hours

123. 5 mL immediately

124. 900 µg = 0.9 mg = child's dose = 0.9 mL

125. 60 mg = child's dose. Each 20-mg dose = 2.5 mL x 3 times a day = 7.5 mL in 24 hours

126. 12.5 mg = child's dose. Each 12.5 mg dose = 0.5 mL

127. 63 mg = child's dose. Each 21-mg dose = 2.1 mL x 3 times a day = 6.3 mL in 24 hours

128. 40 µg = 0.40 mg = child's dose = 0.1 mL

129. 0.1 mL Humulin-R + 0.22 mL Humulin-N = 0.32 mL

130. 0.25 mL @ 07:30 and 16:30

131. 0.08 mL

132. 0.29 mL

133. 0.15 mL

134. 0.3 mL

135. 0.56 mL Lente + 0.1 mL Toronto = 0.66 mL

136. 0.15 mL

137. 0.25 mL NPH + 0.1 mL Toronto = 0.35 mL

138. 0.1 mL

139. 0.8 mL

140. 0.3 mL

141. 10 mL

142. 4 mL

143. 0.5 mL

144. 20 mL

145. 15 mL

146. 7.5 mL

147. 0.2 mL

148. 4 mL

149. Add 0.9 mL hourly or 9.0 mL to 500 mL I.V. N/S

150. Add 0.65 mL hourly or 6.5 mL to 500 mL I.V. N/S

151. Add 0.05 mL hourly or 0.5 mL to 500 mL I.V. N/S

152. Add 0.8 mL hourly or 8 mL to 500 mL I.V. $^2/_3$ & $^1/_3$

153. Add 0.55 mL hourly or 5.5 mL to 500 mL I.V. $^2/_3$ & $^1/_3$

154. Add 10 mL to 500 mL I.V. N/S

155. Add 10 mL to 500 mL I.V. D5W

156. 16.6 = 17 gtts./min

157. 20.8 = 21 gtts./min

158. 12.5 = 13 gtts./min x 1 h, then 25 gtts./min

159. 175 gtts./min

160. 40 gtts./min

161. 30 gtts./min

162. 33 gtts./min x 1 h, then 15 gtts./min

163. 150 gtts./min

164. 7.5 = 8 gtts./min

165. 30 gtts./min

166. 33.3 = 33 gtts./min

167. 20 gtts./min

168. 200 gtts./min x 2 h, then 125 gtts./min

169. 70 gtts./min

170. 40 gtts./min x 3 h, then 50 gtts./min x 20 h

171. 100 or 102 gtts./min

172. 21 gtts./min

173. 42 gtts./min

174. 21 gtts./min x 24 h, then 16 or 17 gtts./min x 10 h

175. 150 gtts./min x 20 min, then 198 or 200 gtts./min

      x 5 h

176. 2 : 25

177. 3 : 20

178. 3 : 4

179. 27 : 100

180. 1 : 400

181. 12.5%

182. 60%

183. 43.75% = 43.8%

184. 44.4%

185. 0.44% = 0.4%

186. 4 mL

187. 50 mL

188. 200 mL

189. 10 mL

190. 10 mL

191. 62.5 mL of solvent is combined with 62.5 mL of 10% stock solution to provide 125 mL of 5% solution.

    62.5 mL + 62.5 mL = 125 mL

192. 83.4 mL of solvent is combined with 416.6 mL of 30% stock solution to provide 500 mL of 25% solution.

    83.4 mL + 416.6 = 500 mL

193. 166.7 mL of solvent is combined with 133.3 mL of 90% stock solution to provide 300 mL of 40% solution.

    166.7 mL + 133.3 mL = 300 mL

194. 500 mL of solvent is combined with 500 mL of 20% stock solution to provide 1 000 mL (1 L) of 10% solution.

    500 mL + 500 mL = 1 000 mL = 1 L

195. 1 200 mL of solvent is combined with 300 mL of 75% stock solution to provide 1 500 mL of 15% solution.

    1 200 mL + 300 mL = 1 500 mL

196. 500 mL

197. 50 mL

198. 1 000 mL

199. 80 mL

200. 3 000 mL

APPENDIX J

Definitions

Ampule (Ampoule)—A sealed glass container.

Base Units—The seven units of measurement from which all other units in the SI system are derived.

BSA—Body surface area.

Capsule—A drug contained within a gelatin-like shell.

Complex fraction—A fraction in which there is a fraction in the numerator, denominator, or both.

CPS—*Compendium of Pharmaceuticals and Specialties*; a reference guide to pharmaceutical products published by the Canadian Pharmaceutical Association.

Decimal number (Decimal fraction)—The result when the numerator of a fraction has been divided by the denominator.

Degree Celsius—The accepted measurement of temperature for SI.

Denominator—The divisor in a fraction; the number below the line.

Diluent—The solution used to dissolve a powder.

Dilution table—A table providing dosage equivalencies for varied amounts of diluent.

Dividend—The number to be divided.

Divisor—The number by which a dividend is divided.

Dosage—The determination and control of the size and number of doses.

Dose—The amount of medication administered at a specific time.

Drop factor—The number of drops per millilitre of fluid administered intravenously.

Elixir—A clear, sweetened, hydroalcoholic liquid, usually containing medicinal substances and taken orally.

Enteric-coated—A coating on tablets used to prevent the release and absorption of a drug until it reaches the intestines.

Extremes—The first and fourth terms of a proportion.

Flow rate—The number of drops per minute a fluid is administered intravenously.

Fraction—The division of a whole number.

Gram—The base unit of mass in the metric system.

Improper fraction—A fraction in which the numerator is equal to or larger than the denominator.

Infusion—The slow introduction of fluid into a vein for therapeutic purposes.

Intramuscular—Into the muscle.

Intravenous—Into the vein.

Invert—To turn upside down or reverse the order of elements.

I.V. push—A small volume of drug injected through a syringe into the bloodstream.

Largest common divisor—The largest number that will divide evenly into the numerator and the denominator.

Lethal dose—A dose that is large enough to result in death.

Litre (Liter)—The base unit of volume in the metric system.

Lowest common denominator—The smallest number into which all denominators found in a group of fractions are divisible.

Maximal dose—The largest dose that can be administered without causing undesirable results.

Means—The second and third terms of a proportion.

Medication order—Instructions written for the preparation and administration of medications.

Metre (Meter)—The base unit of length in the metric system.

Minimal dose—The smallest dose that produces a therapeutic effect.

Mixed number—A fraction preceded by a whole number.

Mole—The base unit of substance in the metric system.

Multiplicand—The number that is to be multiplied.

Multiplier—The number by which another number is to be multiplied.

Nomogram—A graph with several scales arranged so that a straight edge laid on the graph intersects the scales at related values of the variables; the values of any two variables can be used to find the values of the others.

Numerator—The dividend in a fraction; the number above the line.

Parenteral—Administration of medication via any route other than the alimentary canal, such as intravenously, intramuscularly, and subcutaneously.

Percent—The number of hundredths; written as %.

Proper fraction—A fraction in which the numerator is smaller than the denominator.

Proportion—Two ratios of equal value; their relationship is shown through the use of a double colon.

Pure drug—100 parts of a drug.

Ratio—A relationship between two numbers separated by a colon; the expression of a fraction.

Reconstitution—The process of dissolving a powder in a diluent.

Scored tablets—Tablets with indentations allowing for easy division when only part of the medication is to be administered.

SI—The current metric system of measurement used in Canada. It comes from the French name, le Système international d'unités.

Solute—The substance being dissolved.

Solution—A clear, homogenous mixture that results from dissolving one or more substances in a liquid.

Solvent—The liquid used in dissolving a substance.

Stock solution—A pure drug dissolved in a liquid.

Subcutaneous—Into the tissue just below the skin.

Subunits—Units of measurement derived from the SI base units by adding prefixes.

Suspension—A liquid medication in which the drug is not evenly dissolved, generally taken orally.

Syrup—A liquid medication that is sweetened or flavored and taken orally.

Tablets—Drugs compressed into a variety of shapes and colors.

Term—Either of the two numbers in a fraction or ratio.

Therapeutic range—The range of doses, between the minimal and maximal dose, that produces a desired effect.

Toxic dose—A dose that results in a poisonous effect.

Vial—A glass container with a rubber stopper.

APPENDIX K

Common Abbreviations and Symbols Relevant to Dosages and Solutions

@	at
aa or ana	equal parts (of each)
a.c.	before meals
agit.	shake, stir
a.m.	before noon or morning
aq.	water
aq. dist.	distilled water
amp.	ampule
b.i.d.	twice a day
b.i.n.	twice a night
E	with
caps.	capsule
d.	day
D5W	5% dextrose and water solution
D10W	10% dextrose and water solution
dos.	dose
elix.	elixir
et	and
gtt(s).	drop(s)
h	hour
h.s.	bedtime
I.M. or i.m.	intramuscular
I.V.	intravenous
KCl	potassium chloride
L	litre
m. et n.	morning and night
μg or mcg	microgram
mEq	milliequivalents

mg	milligram
$MgSO_4$	magnesium sulphate
mL	millilitre
mol	mole
mmol	millimole
min	minute
n. or nocte	night
N.P.O.	nothing by mouth
N/S	normal saline solution
o.d. or q.d.	every day, once a day
OD	right eye
o.h. or q.h.	every hour
o.m.	every morning
o.n.	every night
OS	left eye
os	mouth
OU	each eye
p.c.	after meals
p.m.	after noon
p.o.	by mouth, orally
p.r.n.	when required
q.	every
q.d.	every day
q.2h	every 2 hours (or any number)
q.i.d.	four times a day
q.o.d.	every other day
R/L	Ringer's lactate solution
s or s.	without
S/L	sublingual
ss or ss	one half
s.o.s.	one dose if necessary
stat.	immediately
subcu. or S.C.	subcutaneous
supp.	suppository
susp.	suspension

syr.	syrup
tab(s).	tablet(s)
t.i.d.	three times a day
t.i.n.	three times a night
Tr. or Tinct.	tincture
troch.	lozenge
ung.	ointment

APPENDIX L

Metric Base Units

Quantity	SI Unit	Symbol
Time	second	s
Electric Current	ampere	A
Thermodynamic temperature	Kelvin	K
Luminous intensity	candela	cd
Length	metre	m
Mass	kilogram	kg
Amount of substance	mole	mol

APPENDIX M

Alternate Formulae for Calculating a Child's Dose

1. *Clark's Rule:*

    This formula compares the weight of the child (in lbs.) to the average weight of an adult (150 lbs.).

    $$\frac{\text{WEIGHT OF CHILD}}{150 \text{ lbs.}} \times \text{ADULT DOSE} = \text{CHILD'S DOSE}$$

    EXAMPLE: The adult dose of pethidine HCl (Demerol) is 50 mg. What is the dose for a child weighing 50 lbs.?

    $$\frac{50 \text{ lbs.}}{150 \text{ lbs.}} \times 50 \text{ mg} =$$

    $$\frac{2\,500 \text{ mg}}{150} \times 16.6 \text{ mg} = 17 \text{ mg}$$

    Child's dose = 17 mg

    NOTE: Round off answers to a whole number for tablets or capsules.

2. *Young's Rule:*

    This formula is used for children 2 to 12 years old.

    $$\frac{\text{AGE}}{\text{AGE} + 12} \times \text{ADULT DOSE} = \text{CHILD'S DOSE}$$

EXAMPLE: The adult dose of cloxacillin sodium (Orbenin) is 500 mg. What is the dose for a child 8 years old?

$$\frac{8}{8 + 12} \times 500 \text{ mg} =$$

$$\frac{8}{20} \times 500 \text{ mg} =$$

$$0.4 \times 500 \text{ mg} = 200 \text{ mg}$$

Child's dose = 200 mg

3. *Fried's Rule:*

This formula is used for children younger than 2 years old.

$$\frac{\text{ADULT DOSE} \times \text{INFANT'S AGE (in months)}}{150 \text{ lbs. (average weight of an adult)}} = \text{INFANT'S DOSE}$$

EXAMPLE: The adult dose of chloral hydrate (Noctec) is 0.5 g. What is the dose for an infant 10 months old?

$$\frac{0.5 \text{ g} \times 10 \text{ months}}{150 \text{ lbs.}} =$$

$$\frac{5.0}{150} = 0.03 \text{ g}$$

Child's dose = 0.03 g

4. *Body Surface Area (BSA)*

This is thought to be the most accurate for calculating pediatric dosages. Body surface area is measured in square metres (m^2). This is measured by using the child's height (cm or ins.) and weight (kg or lbs.) and the West nomogram for BSA .

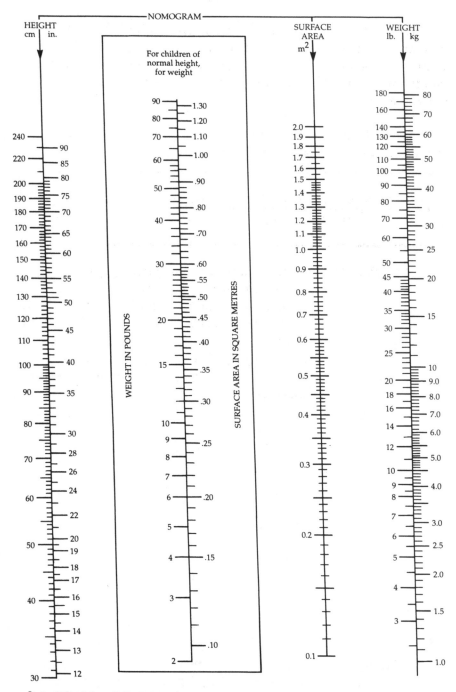

[Modified by C.D. West from data of E. Boyd. From Shirkey, H.C., Drug Therapy. In: *Textbook of Pediatrics*, 9th ed. Nelson, W.E. Vaughn, V.C., III, eds. Philadelphia: W.B. Saunders Co., 1964.]

To use the nomogram, locate the child's height on the left side and the child's weight on the right side of the graph. The point at which a straight line connecting the height and the weight columns intersects the surface area column is the surface area in m².

Varied formulae exist for calculating BSA. The most frequently used formulae are given.

$$\frac{\text{Body surface area of child (m}^2) \times \text{Adult dose}}{1.73 \ (m^2) \ (\text{average adult BSA})} = \text{Child's dose}$$

EXAMPLE #1: The physician orders diphenhydramine HCl (Benadryl) I.M. for a child whose height is 116 cm and weight is 19 kg. Calculate this child's dose if the adult dose is 50 mg.

The first step is to obtain the body surface area of this child. Refer to the West nomogram.

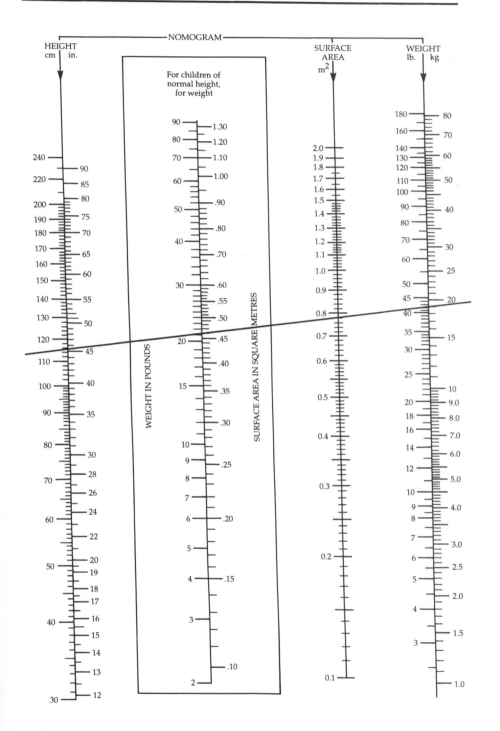

HEIGHT
cm | in.

For children of
normal height,
for weight

WEIGHT IN POUNDS

SURFACE AREA IN SQUARE METRES

SURFACE
AREA
m²

WEIGHT
lb. | kg

*The nomogram indicates that the surface area for a child
whose height is 116 cm and weight is 19 kg is 0.78 m².*

$$\frac{\text{Body surface area of child (m}^2)\ \times\ \text{Adult dose}}{1.73\ (\text{m}^2)\ (\text{average adult BSA})} = \text{Child's dose}$$

$$\frac{0.78\ \text{m}^2\ \times\ 50\ \text{mg}}{1.73\ \text{m}^2} =$$

$$\frac{39}{1.73} = 22.5\ \text{mg}$$

Child's dose = 22.5 mg

The physician may order a child's dose by dosage/m². The following formula can be used for such an order.

$$\text{Body surface area of a child (m}^2)\ \times\ \text{Dose/m}^2\ =\ \text{Child's dose}$$

EXAMPLE #2: The physician orders phenobarbital sodium (Luminal) 60 mg/m² of body surface p.o. for a child whose height is 90 cm and whose weight is 14 kg. Calculate this child's dose.

The first step is to obtain the body surface area of this child. Refer to the West nomogram.

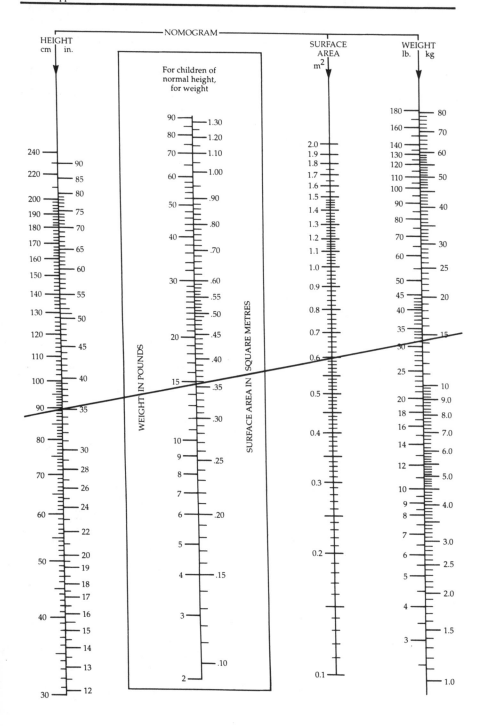

The nomogram indicates that the surface area for a child whose height is 90 cm and weight is 14 kg is 0.6 m².

Body surface area of a child (m^2) x Dose/m^2 = Child's dose

$$0.6 \, m^2 \times 60 \, mg/m^2 = 36 \, mg$$

$$Child's \, dose = 36 \, mg$$

APPENDIX N

Insulins

Product Name and Action	Type	Species Source-Structure
SHORT-ACTING		
Insulin-Toronto	Regular	Beef/Pork
Iletin Regular	Regular	Beef/Pork
Semilente Insulin	Semilente	Beef/Pork
Semilente Iletin	Semilente	Beef/Pork
Iletin II	Regular	Pork
Velosulin	Regular	Pork
Novolin-Toronto	Regular	Human-Semisynthetic
Humulin-R	Regular	Human-Biosynthetic
Velosulin Human	Regular	Human-Semisynthetic
INTERMEDIATE-ACTING		
Lente Insulin	Lente	Beef/Pork
Lente Iletin	Lente	Beef/Pork
NPH Insulin	NPH	Beef/Pork
NPH Iletin	NPH	Beef/Pork
Iletin II Lente	Lente	Pork
Iletin II NPH	NPH	Pork
Insulatard	NPH	Pork
Novolin-Lente	Lente	Human-Semisynthetic
Humulin-L	Lente	Human-Biosynthetic
Novolin-NPH	NPH	Human-Semisynthetic
Humulin-N	NPH	Human-Biosynthetic
Insulatard Human	NPH	Human-Semisynthetic

Product Name and Action	Type	Species Source-Structure
LONG ACTING		
Novolin-Ultralente	Ultralente	Human-Semisynthetic
Humulin-U	Ultralente	Human-Biosynthetic
Ultralente Insulin	Ultralente	Beef/Pork
Ultralente Iletin	Ultralente	Beef/Pork
Protamine Zinc Insulin	PZI	Beef/Pork
Protamine Zinc Iletin	PZI	Beef/Pork
MIXTURES		
Mixtard (intermediate-acting)	Regular 30% NPH 70%	Pork
Initard (intermediate-acting)	Regular 50% NPH 50%	Pork
Mixtard Human (intermediate-acting)	Regular 30% NPH 70%	Human-Semisynthetic
Initard Human (intermediate-acting)	Regular 50% NPH 50%	Human-Semisynthetic
Novolin-30/70	Regular 30% NPH 70%	Human-Semisynthetic

APPENDIX O

Equivalencies Relevant to the Three Systems of Measurement

Liquid Measure

Metric	Approx. Apothecary Equivalents
1 000 mL	1 quart
750 mL	1 1/2 pints
500 mL	1 pint
250 mL	8 fluid ounces
30 mL	1 fluid ounce
4 mL	1 fluid dram
1 mL	15 minims

Weight

Metric	Approx. Apothecary Equivalents
30 g	1 ounce
15 g	4 drams
10 g	2 1/2 drams
2 g	30 grains (1/2 dram)
1 g	15 grains
30 mg	1/2 grain
4 mg	1/15 grain
1 mg	1/60 grain
0.1 mg	1/600 grain

| Metric | | | Approx. Apothecary Equivalents |
Liquid	Weight	Height	
5 mL	5 g		1 teaspoon
15 mL	15 g		3 teaspoons = 1 tablespoon
237 mL	240 g		1 cup = 16 tablespoons
473 mL	480 g		2 cups = 1 pint
946 mL	960 g		4 cups = 2 pints = 1 quart
		2.54 cm	1 inch
	1 kg		2.2 pounds

APPENDIX P

Summary of Formulae Outlined in Chapters 4 to 8

$$\frac{\text{DOSE DESIRED}}{\text{DOSE ON HAND}} \times \text{DRUG FORM} = \text{AMOUNT TO ADMINISTER}$$

The *dose desired* is the dose of medication to be administered.
The *dose on hand* is the dose of medication available.
The *drug form* is how the medication is supplied. It is equivalent to the *dose on hand*.

1. *A general formula for calculating medications.*

$$\text{DRUG DOSE} \times \text{CHILD'S WEIGHT} = \text{CHILD'S DOSE}$$
$$\text{(in mg/kg)} \qquad \text{(in kilograms)}$$

2. *A formula for a child's dose.*

$$\frac{\text{DROP FACTOR} \times \text{RATE PER HOUR}}{60 \text{ MINUTES/HOUR}} = \text{FLOW RATE (gtts./min)}$$
$$\text{(gtts./mL)} \qquad \text{(mL/h)}$$

3. *A general formula for calculating flow rates.*

$$\text{DROP FACTOR} \times \text{MILLILITRES PER MINUTE} = \text{FLOW RATE}$$

(gtts./mL)   (mL/min)   (gtts./min)

4. *A metric standard formula for flow rates.*

DRUG : SOLVENT : : PERCENT : 100

5. *A formula for calculating percentage concentration.*

$$\frac{\text{DESIRED STRENGTH}}{\text{AVAILABLE STRENGTH}} = \frac{\text{AMOUNT TO USE}}{\text{AMOUNT TO MAKE}}$$

6. *A formula for diluting stock solutions.*

Desired Strength : Available Strength : : Amt. to Use : Amt. to Make

7. *A formula using proportions for diluting stock solutions.*

Bibliography

Boyer, M.J. *Math for Nurses: A Pocket Guide to Dosage Calculation and Drug Preparation.* Philadelphia, Pennsylvania: J.P. Lippincott, 1987.

Compendium of Pharmaceuticals and Specialties. Ottawa, Ontario: Canadian Pharmaceutical Association, 22nd ed., 1987.

Curren, A.M., L.D. Munday, *Math for Meds: A Programmed Text of Dosages and Solutions.* Willowdale, Ontario: McAinsh & Co., Ltd., 1986.

Dickson, T.R. *Introduction to Chemistry.* Toronto, Ontario: John Wiley & Sons, Inc., 1987.

Miller, B.F., C.B. Keane, *Encyclopedia and Dictionary of Medicine, Nursing, and Allied Health.* Toronto, Ontario: W.B. Saunders Co., 3rd ed., 1983.

Olsen, J.L., L.J. Ablon, A.P. Giangrasso, H. Siner-Weissman, *Medical Dosage Calculations.* Toronto, Ontario: Addison-Wesley Publishing Company, 4th ed., 1987.

S.I. Manual in Health Care. Toronto: Government of Ontario. 2nd ed., 1983.

Whisler, B.L. *Mathematics for Health Professionals.* Belmont, California: Wadsworth Health Services Division, 1985.

Woodrow, R. *Essentials of Pharmacology for Health Occupations.* Toronto, Ontario: John Wiley & Sons, Inc., 1987.